Secrets of a Long and Healthy Life

By

ALICE DEE

ALICE DEE

First Edition

Copyright © 2024 Alice Dee

All rights reserved. This book or any portion thereof
may not be reproduced or used in any manner whatsoever
without the express written permission of the author
except for the use of brief quotations in a book review.

www.RawFromTheGarden.com

www.NutritionalHealer.com

www.PeakPerformanceDiet.com

www.TheFoodForestGuide.com

ISBN: 9798876485052

DEDICATION

This book is gratefully dedicated to the love of my life.

ACKNOWLEDGEMENTS

I wish to acknowledge the inspiration of my unusually long-lived mother who chose to follow a different and healthier diet as a teenager and has since outlived both of her parents and her brother by 30 years or more.

TABLE OF CONTENTS

PREFACE

In the ever-evolving study of life, where the pursuit of health and longevity stands as a timeless endeavor, I am delighted to welcome you to "Secrets of a Long and Healthy Life." As the author of this exploration into the secrets of vibrant well-being, it is both an honor and a privilege to guide you on a path of healthful transformation through the upcoming pages.

As a passionate advocate for holistic living and natural nutrition, I have dedicated my life to understanding the profound connections between lifestyle choices, diet, and the pursuit of a flourishing existence. This book is the culmination of decades of research, personal experiences, and an unwavering commitment to unraveling the mysteries that surround the art of aging gracefully.

Not just a compilation of facts and figures; this book extends a heartfelt invitation to reconsider your relationship with time, health, and the choices that shape your everyday life. Drawing from the wisdom of experts, scientific studies, personal experiences, and the testimonies of other individuals who have embraced the tenets of well-being expounded herein, each chapter is crafted with the intent of empowering you to make informed decisions that resonate with the rhythms of your own life and achieving its maximum extension.

Throughout these pages, you will encounter the transformative potential of a natural diet and learn about a science-based dietary paradigm that serves as the cornerstone of our study together. Beyond the realms of nutrition, we will explore the detailed interplay of exercise, sleep, stress management, and social connections, understanding how each element contributes to the goal of maximizing our longevity.

As you join me in this exploration, my hope is to inspire you not only to adopt healthier habits but to foster a mindset that embraces the richness of life in all its dimensions. "Secrets of a Long and Healthy Life" is an invitation to engage with your well-being on a profound level, to embrace life's journey with curiosity, and to savor the discoveries that unfold along the way.

I extend my deepest gratitude to you, dear reader, for embarking on this odyssey with me. May the insights within these pages be a guiding light on your path toward a life that is not only long but filled with good health, vibrancy, purpose, meaning, and happiness.

To your health!

Alice Dee

INTRODUCTION

INTRODUCTION

In the hustle and bustle of our modern lives, where the pace seems ever quickening and demands relentlessly mount, the pursuit of longevity and well-being has become a paramount concern for many people.

"Secrets of a Long and Healthy Life" will take you on a fascinating study into the heart of sustainable living and the practical and well-tested methods you can use to extend your lifetime. Reading it will help you gradually unravel the secrets to a life rich in both years and vitality from the irrefutable science-based facts and logic presented in this book.

As you delve into the pages of this exploration, it will become clear that the fountain of youth is not a mythical spring, but a dynamic amalgamation of mindful choices, nourishing practices, and a profound understanding of the complex relationship between our bodies and the world around us.

Far beyond the constraints of mere genetic predispositions, this book illuminates the potent influence of environment and nutrition on our overall well-being. It thus offers a blueprint for those who seek not only longevity but a life teeming with energy, purpose, and joy.

Our journey together begins by peeling back the layers of conventional wisdom surrounding nutrition, where the cornerstone of our quest lies in the transformative potential of a natural diet best suited to our physiology and primate ancestry.

See through the healthful lens of wholesome, unprocessed foods, you will explore the profound impact that mindful eating can have on the body's interconnected physiology and its associated mental status. This essential understanding will lay the groundwork for the sustained health and vitality of your body and mind.

Yet, this book is not a mere dietary manual. It is instead a comprehensive guide that navigates the holistic terrain of a well-lived existence to give you concrete advice you can use to lengthen your life while enjoying better overall health.

From the rhythmic cadence of exercise and the rejuvenating embrace of quality sleep to the resilience cultivated through stress management and the profound influence of social connections, each chapter unfurls another layer of the foundation that underlies a healthy life, revealing the interconnected threads that form the fabric of a flourishing being.

As you traverse the chapters of this book, you may need to confront harmful habits and learn to embrace the importance of regular health check-ups. You will also explore why engaging in a lifelong learning program can help keep the mind sharp and able to focus.

The narrative of this book is woven with the golden threads of positivity, purpose, and fulfillment, recognizing their integral roles in the pursuit of a life that transcends the mere accumulation of years.

As you read it, keep in mind that this book is not a promise of immortality but a practical roadmap for those seeking a life imbued with well-being, resilience, and fulfillment. It beckons you now to embark on a path of transformation, inviting you to explore the multifaceted facets of health and longevity.

So, let us turn the pages together, as we unravel the secrets that pave the way to a life well-lived, a life that dances gracefully and healthily through the sands of time.

Understanding the Foundations of Longevity

As you start to study longevity, it is essential to establish a foundational understanding of the many factors that help shape a healthy and enduring life.

Countless studies from reputable authorities in the fields of medicine, nutrition, and wellness converge to emphasize the pivotal role that lifestyle choices, especially diet, play in the quest for longevity.

In the pursuit of longevity, it also becomes evident that genetics, though playing a role, does not wield an absolute dominion over our fate. This concept of epigenetics underscores the empowering notion that our choices have the potential to shape the trajectory of our well-being.

Our exploration into the foundations of longevity, therefore, extends beyond mere theoretical conjecture. It is rooted in a wealth of scientific research and observations drawn from real-world examples.

In the pages that follow, you will be introduced to the core principles that underpin your chances of living a long and healthy life, drawing inspiration from the wisdom of those who have dedicated their lives to unraveling the secrets of aging with grace and vitality.

The Role of Lifestyle Choices

In our quest for longevity, the profound impact of lifestyle choices becomes an undeniable focal point. Grounded in scientific research and bolstered by the insights of experts, this book will shed light on the transformative potential of conscious eating decisions, with a particular emphasis on advocating a raw plant-based diet based on that of our closets primate relatives as a cornerstone for optimal health and enduring vitality.

Beyond nutrition, the role of getting adequate sleep and physical activity in promoting longevity is indisputable. Integrating regular exercise into our lives becomes a complementary dimension to a plant-based diet, fortifying the body against the degenerative effects of aging. Establishing and cultivating positive relationships also plays a substantial part in extending lifespans.

As you navigate through the following chapters, it is this foundation of nutritional wisdom, empirical evidence, and the integration of holistic lifestyle factors that will guide your exploration into the science of promoting longevity.

CHAPTER 1: THE POWER OF NUTRITION

INTRODUCTION

When it comes to exploring the topics of extending health and longevity, the compass pointing towards optimal well-being inevitably directs us to the profound influence of nutrition. This chapter dives deep into the details of optimal dietary choices, unveiling the notable impact of nutrition on our health and longevity.

As you start to understand the significance of diet to your success as a living being, it becomes apparent that our food choices are not mere sustenance but a potent determinant of the quality and duration of our lives.

As you read through the pages that follow, do your best to immerse yourself in and accept how important good nutrition is to your well-being. You will also discover the transformative potential of a raw plant-based diet in nourishing our bodies for greater vitality and longevity.

Unveiling the Importance of Diet to Health

Nutrition, as championed by renowned experts in the field, serves as a key cornerstone in the pursuit of a long and healthy life. Dr. David L. Katz, in "Disease-Proof: Slash Your Risk of Heart Disease, Cancer, Diabetes, and More—by 80 Percent," unravels the detailed connection between dietary habits and the prevention of chronic diseases.[1]

Furthermore, Dr. Caldwell Esselstyn, a leading figure in the field of preventative cardiology and the plant-based nutrition movement, asserts in "Prevent and Reverse Heart Disease" that adopting a diet centered on unprocessed plant foods can not only prevent but also reverse heart disease, demonstrating the health-transforming potential of plant-powered nutrition.[2]

---

[1] David L. Katz, Stacey Colino, "Disease-Proof: Slash Your Risk of Heart Disease, Cancer, Diabetes, and More—by 80 Percent," Hudson Street Press, 2013.

His work emphasizes the remarkable capacity of plant-based diets to not only prevent but also reverse heart disease, advocating for a comprehensive shift in dietary habits for sustained well-being.[3]

Dr. Esselstyn's pioneering research extends beyond heart health to illuminate the broader implications for longevity. It demonstrates that a plant-based diet not only prevents and can help reverse heart disease and other vascular issues, but it contributes substantially to overall well-being, offering a roadmap for nurturing the body towards enduring health.[4]

Furthermore, Dr. Dean Ornish, a clinical professor of medicine at the University of California, emphasizes that lifestyle changes, including dietary modifications, can influence the expression of genes related to health and longevity.[5]

Dr. Michael Greger, in "How Not to Die," also explores the multifaceted benefits of plant-based nutrition in great detail, emphasizing how such choices contribute not only to individual health but also to broader environmental sustainability.[6] Dr. Greger also stresses the health benefits derived from dietary diversity, highlighting how consuming different plant foods contributes unique sets of nutrients that collectively foster optimal well-being.[7]

In essence, by adopting a whole-food, plant-centric diet, you can embark on a transformative path to better health that not only nourishes your body but serves as a shield against the chronic ailments that often accompany the passage of time.

Exploring the Benefits of a Living Foods Diet

Now it's time to explore the details of the optimal nourishment for a long and healthy life. This study inevitably leads us to expound the many benefits

---

[2] Caldwell B. Esselstyn Jr., "Prevent and Reverse Heart Disease: The Revolutionary, Scientifically Proven, Nutrition-Based Cure," Avery, 2007.

[3] Caldwell B. Esselstyn Jr., ibid.

[4] Caldwell B. Esselstyn Jr., ibid.

[5] Dean Ornish, "Changing Your Lifestyle Can Change Your Genes - for Good," *The Washington Post*, 2018.

[6] Michael Greger, Gene Stone, "How Not to Die: Discover the Foods Scientifically Proven to Prevent and Reverse Disease," Flatiron Books, 2015.

[7] Michael Greger, Gene Stone, ibid.

of a raw plant-based diet, a nutritional paradigm that emerges as a potent catalyst for sustaining vitality and resilience throughout your life.

The concept of consuming a raw plant-based diet consisting solely of whole and uncooked living foods derived from plants extends beyond mere sufficient sustenance; it embodies a philosophy of nourishing the body at its most elemental and optimal level.

Basically, since no other creature cooks their food and heating food significantly reduces its nutritional value and enzymatic content, the fact that eating plant-derived foods in their natural raw state is good for us and helps us live longer makes remarkable sense as I have written about in detail in my book "Why Raw Vegan?" [8]

Furthermore, the works of Dr. Gabriel Cousens, particularly in "Rainbow Green Live-Food Cuisine," expound in great detail upon the rejuvenating qualities of raw plant-based diets. In his books, Dr. Cousens elucidates how a diet rich in enzymes, vitamins, and phytonutrients derived from uncooked plant sources can invigorate our bodies, thereby bolstering our defenses against the impacts of aging and environmental stressors.[9]

The Value of Periodic Fasting

Fasting consists of refraining from eating for some period of time. Fasts can last from several hours to 40 days in duration, although fasts longer than a week are generally best done under medical supervision. Some fasts might include drinking juices and broths, while others only involve drinking water.

Dr. Valter D. Longo, a renowned longevity researcher and director of the Longevity Institute at the University of Southern California, underscores the significance of dietary interventions like periodic fasting in promoting healthy aging. His groundbreaking research that was published in the journal *Cell Metabolism* illuminates the profound impact of occasional fasting on cellular regeneration and the mitigation of age-related diseases.[10]

This highlights the notion that the way we nourish our bodies, particularly

---

[8] Alice Dee, "Why Raw Vegan?", Raw From the Garden Press, 2017.

[9] Gabriel Cousens, "Rainbow Green Live-Food Cuisine," North Atlantic Books, 2003.

[10] Valter D. Longo, "Fasting: Molecular Mechanisms and Clinical Applications," *Cell Metabolism* 2014.

through consciously choosing what to eat and when to eat or not to eat, can wield transformative effects on the very fabric of our health.

Nourishing Your Body for Longevity

As you continue this exploration into the role of nutrition in promoting a lengthy lifespan, the underlying premise is clear: nourishing your body for longevity often requires a profound shift in dietary habits from what you may be used to.

The Blue Zones, areas of the world known for exceptional longevity, consistently feature plant-based diets as a common thread among their inhabitants.[11] The meticulous research of Dan Buettner and his team into these Blue Zones highlights commonalities in the habits of these long-lived populations, such as plant-based diets, strong social connections, and regular physical activity.[12] Their findings serve as a testament to the notable impact of lifestyle choices in fostering resilience and well-being throughout the aging process.

For example, the Okinawan diet, celebrated for its role in the longevity of the Okinawan population in Japan, aligns closely with the principles of a raw plant-based approach. This diet, characterized by a predominantly plant-based and nutrient-dense intake, has been associated with an unusually high number of centenarians in the region.[13]

The Okinawan diet is the traditional eating pattern of the people of the Japanese island of Okinawa. This diet provides a compelling real-world example blueprint for nourishing the body towards a ripe old age that was documented extensively in "The Okinawa Program" by Bradley J. Willcox, D. Craig Willcox, and Makoto Suzuki.

Rich in vegetables, legumes, and sweet potatoes, with minimal meat consumption, this diet has been associated with exceptional longevity and a lower prevalence of age-related diseases.[14] This dietary pattern is unusually rich in nutrients and antioxidants, and it exemplifies the potential of a plant-

---

[11] Dan Buettner, "The Blue Zones: Lessons for Living Longer From the People Who've Lived the Longest," National Geographic Society, 2008

[12] Dan Buettner, ibid.

[13] Bradley J. Willcox, D. Craig Willcox, Makoto Suzuki, "The Okinawa Program: How the World's Longest-Lived People Achieve Everlasting Health," Clarkson Potter, 2001.

[14] Bradley J. Willcox, D. Craig Willcox, Makoto Suzuki, ibid.

centric approach in fostering a long and vibrant life.

The Role of Nutrition in Immune Function

A raw plant-based diet is inherently rich in essential nutrients, which aligns seamlessly with the principles of how to sustain a strong immune system that paves the way for a resilient and enduring life. In his book "Super Immunity," Dr. Joel Fuhrman introduces the concept of nutrient density as a critical factor in supporting the immune system and overall health.[15]

Furthermore, real-world examples from populations following predominantly plant-based diets, as highlighted in Dr. T. Colin Campbell's "The China Study," underscore the broader implications for health and longevity.[16] These examples illuminate the potential for embracing the principles of a raw plant-based diet not only to prevent diseases but to nurture our bodies towards a life of enduring vibrancy.

Dr. David L. Katz, a pioneer in preventive medicine, has extensively researched the strong connection between dietary choices and disease prevention as explained in his book in "Disease-Proof: Slash Your Risk of Heart Disease, Cancer, Diabetes, and More—by 80 Percent." His compelling research emphasizes the strong impact of a nutrient-rich diet in slashing the risk of heart disease, cancer, diabetes, and other chronic ailments.[17] This underscores the pivotal role that nutrition plays in shaping our health destinies over the long term.

Furthermore, numerous epidemiological studies, including the especially well-known Nurses' Health Study and the Health Professionals Follow-up Study, consistently highlight the correlation between plant-based diets and a reduced risk of chronic diseases.[18] These findings underscore the importance of shifting our dietary focus towards whole, plant-based foods for optimal health and longevity.

---

[15] Joel Fuhrman, "Super Immunity: The Essential Nutrition Guide for Boosting Your Body's Defenses to Live Longer, Stronger, and Disease Free," HarperOne, 2012.

[16] T. Colin Campbell, Thomas M. Campbell II, "The China Study: Revised and Expanded Edition," BenBella Books, 2016.

[17] David L. Katz, Stacey Colino, "Disease-Proof: Slash Your Risk of Heart Disease, Cancer, Diabetes, and More—by 80 Percent," Hudson Street Press, 2013.

[18] Frank B. Hu, Teresa T. Fung, et al., "Dietary Patterns and the Risk of Coronary Heart Disease in Women," *Archives of Internal Medicine*, 2001.

Basically, the strong link between a robust immune system and longevity becomes increasingly evident as you review the science on the subject, further reinforcing the benefits of nourishing our bodies with plant-centric nutrition.

The Mediterranean Paradigm

The Mediterranean diet is renowned for its emphasis on plant-based foods, healthy fats, and lean proteins, stands out among modern human diets as an improvement in the realm of heart-healthy nutrition compared to poor diets heavily laden with cooked fast and processed foods. The Mediterranean diet notably focuses on fruits, vegetables, whole grains, and healthy fats, and it has been extensively studied for its role in promoting heart health and longevity.

For example, the PREDIMED trial led by Dr. Ramón Estruch showcases the Mediterranean diet's remarkable ability to reduce cardiovascular events and promote overall well-being.[19] This dietary paradigm reinforces the idea that incorporating plant-based elements into our daily nutrition can yield profound health benefits. Furthermore, Dr. Ancel Keys, a pioneer in nutritional research, has underscored the myriad benefits of this dietary pattern.[20]

These findings lay a foundation for our exploration into the power of nutrition to shape our health destinies. As you continue to explore nutrition's importance to health and longevity, the evidence will become very clear: your dietary choices are not only about satisfying hunger but also about laying the groundwork for a vibrant and enduring life.

BENEFITS OF A RAW FOOD DIET

As you further your exploration of nutrition's life-transforming potential here, the spotlight now turns toward a dietary paradigm that resonates as a paradigm of vitality - the raw plant-based diet. Beyond mere sustenance, this section explains the myriad benefits that unfold when we embrace the

---

[19] Ramón Estruch, et al., "Primary Prevention of Cardiovascular Disease with a Mediterranean Diet Supplemented with Extra-Virgin Olive Oil or Nuts," *The New England Journal of Medicine*, 2018.
[20] Ramón Estruch, et al., "Primary Prevention of Cardiovascular Disease with a Mediterranean Diet Supplemented with Extra-Virgin Olive Oil or Nuts," *The New England Journal of Medicine*, 2018.

purity and vibrancy of uncooked, plant-centric nutrition.

The principles of the previous approaches to health through diet apply and extend seamlessly to a raw plant-based diet. This natural and healthful dietary pattern amplifies the benefits of unprocessed, nutrient-dense foods in promoting cardiovascular and general well-being.

Unlocking the Transformative Potential

Dr. Gabriel Cousens, in "Rainbow Green Live-Food Cuisine," elevates the discourse on raw plant-based nutrition, emphasizing its potential to invigorate our bodies.

As he promotes the consumption of live and enzymatically-rich plant foods, Dr. Cousens explores how a raw plant-based diet can enhance vitality, foster mental clarity, and fortify our immune systems.[21] This perspective opens a gateway to understanding the profound impact of uncooked, whole foods on our holistic well-being.

A core basis for these claims centers on the facts that the vitamin C responsible for optimal immune system functioning, as well as the ephemeral B vitamins that boost energy levels and mental functioning are amply present in raw plant foods but are destroyed by the high temperatures that cooking generally involves.

As you continue to explore the topic of nourishment for longevity, the allure of a raw plant-based diet will continue to beckon. This approach not only honors the wisdom of ancestral diets that fostered enduring health but also aligns with contemporary scientific research, offering a comprehensive and transformative path toward optimal health.

The Therapeutic Potential of Raw Juices

The emphasis on unprocessed and uncooked plant-derived foods as a means of promoting health is a hallmark of the raw food movement.

One notable proponent of this dietary approach is Dr. Max Gerson, a prominent figure in alternative cancer therapies. He expounds upon the therapeutic potential of raw plant-derived juices in treating cancer in his book "A Cancer Therapy: Results of 50 Cases."

---

[21] Gabriel Cousens, "Rainbow Green Live-Food Cuisine," North Atlantic Books, 2003.

Although his work is considered controversial by some health practitioners not familiar with the remarkable healing potential of raw plant food and juices, his remarkable success in treating cancer cases underscores the healing properties of raw plant-based nutrition.[22]

Nutrient Density and Cellular Rejuvenation

Dr. Joel Fuhrman, a leading advocate for plant-based nutrition, introduces us to the concept of nutrient density in "Super Immunity." His research highlights the exceptional nutritional value found in raw, plant-based foods, emphasizing their ability to enhance immune function and promote cellular health.[23]

Additional real-world examples, such as the work of Dr. Colin Campbell in "The China Study," showcase populations where plant-based diets contribute to enhanced health and longevity.[24]

These examples underscore the notion that embracing the principles of a raw plant-based diet aligns not only with individual well-being but with a broader potential for societal health transformation. This research also positions a raw plant-based diet as a formidable strategy for fortifying the body against the impacts of aging and environmental stressors.

A Nutritional Approach to Longevity

When on a quest for greater longevity, studying nutrition should take center stage, and the composition of your diet will serve as a pivotal instrument in creating a life filled with vitality. This section has explained the principles of nourishing your body for enduring health, with a particular focus on the merits of consuming a raw plant-based diet.

The holistic approach of a raw plant-based diet is not just about what we eat; it extends to how we view our relationship with food. Embracing this nutritional paradigm involves recognizing the interconnectedness of our choices — from the nutrients we consume to the impact on our

---

[22] Max Gerson, "A Cancer Therapy: Results of 50 Cases," Totality Books, 1958.

[23] Joel Fuhrman, "Super Immunity: The Essential Nutrition Guide for Boosting Your Body's Defenses to Live Longer, Stronger, and Disease Free," HarperOne, 2012.

[24] T. Colin Campbell, Thomas M. Campbell II, "The China Study: Revised and Expanded Edition," BenBella Books, 2016.

environment.

The path toward optimal health thus welcomes you to embrace the principles of a raw plant-based diet, recognizing it as a cornerstone for the nourishment of our bodies and the cultivation of longevity.

As you explore the topic of nutrition further in the coming sections of this chapter, keep in mind that the many benefits of a raw plant-based diet offer you a transformative path towards enhanced vitality and enduring health.

Gaining this essential understanding invites you to embrace the natural simplicity and vibrancy of uncooked, plant-centric nutrition as a cornerstone for your optimal well-being.

INSIGHTS FROM ANCESTRAL AND PRIMATE DIETS

In the quest for an optimal diet that harmonizes with our physiological makeup, peering into the nutritional habits of our ancestors and our closest great ape relatives, the chimpanzees and bonobos, unveils compelling insights.

Driven by science and a profound understanding of evolutionary biology, this exploration sheds light on the evolutionary path that has shaped our digestive systems and nutritional needs.

The Ancestral Echo: A Glimpse into Primate Diets

Chimpanzees and bonobos both share a common ancestor with humans that consumed a plant-based diet. These extant great ape cousins offer a lens into the natural and raw plant-based dietary patterns that also sustained the vast majority of our ancestors' evolutionary journey dating well back into the Pliocene Era millions of years ago.[25]

Dr. Richard Wrangham, a prominent primatologist, emphasizes that the majority of the diet of wild chimpanzees comprises plant-based foods, with raw fruits and leafy greens dominating their diets that is supplemented by some nuts, seeds, and flowers. [26]

---

[25] Alice Dee, "The Pliocene Diet: A Guide to Healthy Ancestral Eating", Raw From the Garden Press, 2023.

[26] Richard Wrangham, "Catching Fire: How Cooking Made Us Human," Basic Books, 2009.

As a result, the primate diet approach, with its recommended ratio of 50 percent fruit, 40 percent greens, and 10 percent other plant-based foods, becomes a scientifically informed template for the ideal human diet. Such a dietary approach harmonizes with the physiological digestive similarities we share with our Pliocene Era ancestors and with modern day chimpanzees and bonobos who currently consumed a plant-based diet.

Our primate kin also showcase the significance of nutrient-rich diversity in their diets, incorporating a spectrum of fruits, greens, nuts, and seeds into their diet. The 50-40-10 ratio instinctively chosen by those living primates mostly closely related to humans naturally mirrors this diversity while focusing largely on nutrient dense fruits and greens.

This becomes a science-backed prescription for crafting plates for humans that resonate best with our evolutionary heritage. The primate diet thus accurately informs us of what an optimal raw plant-based diet should consist of, further emphasizing the centrality of fruits and greens to ideal human nutrition.

In your path toward optimal health and longevity, embracing a raw plant-based diet thus echoes the dietary patterns etched in the evolutionary fabric of our primate heritage.

The Fiber Connection: An Evolutionary Legacy

Dietary fiber is abundant in fruits, greens, and other plant-based foods. This important dietary component forms a linchpin in the instinctive nutritional choices of our primate counterparts, and should also be strategically considered in a well-constructed human diet.

Drawing on decades of his extensive nutritional research, Dr. T. Colin Campbell underscores the importance of fiber in maintaining gut health, regulating blood sugar levels, and fostering a thriving microbial ecosystem within our digestive tract. [27]

His findings align seamlessly with a primate dietary approach centered on fruits and greens that results in a diet naturally rich in plant-derived fiber that keep our human digestive systems healthy and flowing properly.

---

[27] T. Colin Campbell, Howard Jacobson, "Whole: Rethinking the Science of Nutrition," BenBella Books, 2013

Raw Nutrition: An Evolutionary Blueprint

The dietary habits of chimpanzees and bonobos who generally consume only raw plant-based foods when living wild should prompt a sensible reflection on the benefits of uncooked plant-derived nutrition for humans.

For example, Dr. Jane Goodall's pioneering primatology research consistently highlights the extensive consumption of raw fruits and leafy vegetation by wild chimpanzees.[28]

This resonates with the ideal 50-40-10 primate dietary ratio, where 90 percent of a typical wild chimp's diet comprises raw fruits and greens, reflecting an evolutionary blueprint that aligns well with our own human physiology.

As you explore the core science-based principles of the ideal diet for your physiological adaptations and learn how to integrate that information into your modern life, you will not only start to align with your evolutionary roots but also nourish your body in a way that echoes the wisdom of nature itself.

---

[28] Jane Goodall, "In the Shadow of Man," Houghton Mifflin, 1971.

CHAPTER 2: THE BALANCED PLATE

INTRODUCTION

When it comes to enhancing longevity, the arrangement of our daily sustenance emerges as a key factor, strongly shaping the harmonious interplay of health and well-being. This chapter is a voyage into the art of crafting a balanced plate, a canvas upon which the brushstrokes of nutrient-rich abundance and plant-based vitality come to life.

As we explore the foundational elements of a raw plant-based diet, we will delve into the proportions and varieties that compose the optimal composition for a plate that nourishes the body and nurtures longevity.

Dr. Joel Fuhrman, in "Eat to Live," illuminates the principles of a nutrient-rich diet as the cornerstone of optimal health.[29] The first section of this chapter will cover the essential building blocks of an ideal diet, emphasizing the importance of selecting foods not only for their caloric content but, more importantly, for their nutritional density. Scientific insights and real-world examples will guide us as we understand the transformative potential inherent in adopting a diet rich in vitamins, minerals, and phytonutrients.

The vibrant hues of fruits and greens beckon us towards a nutritional palette conducive to good health and vitality. Dr. Michael Greger, in "How Not to Die," synthesizes extensive research to underscore the unparalleled benefits of incorporating fruits and greens in abundance.[30]

Drawing inspiration from this nutritional wisdom, we will explore the dynamic interplay between fruits and greens, understanding how this duo contributes to optimal digestion, cellular rejuvenation, and immune resilience. Real-world examples from traditional diets and modern nutritional science will illuminate the bountiful spectrum of possibilities a plant-based plate can offer.

---

[29] Joel Fuhrman, "Eat to Live: The Amazing Nutrient-Rich Program for Fast and Sustained Weight Loss," Little, Brown and Company, 2003.
[30] Michael Greger, Gene Stone, "How Not to Die: Discover the Foods Scientifically Proven to Prevent and Reverse Disease," Flatiron Books, 2015.

Creating a balanced plate consistent with our ancestral dietary wisdom does extend somewhat beyond the fruits and greens that form its bulk. This invites the harmonious and more modest inclusion of vegetables, whole grains, legumes, nuts, and seeds into the diet. Dr. T. Colin Campbell, in "Whole: Rethinking the Science of Nutrition," guides us through the comprehensive benefits of incorporating these diverse elements in a plant-based diet.[31]

From the fiber-rich embrace of vegetables to the satiating power of whole grains, added to the protein-packed potency of legumes, nuts, and seeds, this section will illuminate the multifaceted advantages of creating a sampling of nutrient-rich diversity on our plates.

The principles of Dr. Joel Fuhrman's "Nutritarian" approach will be introduced to serve as an example of a plant-based dietary pattern for crafting plates that prioritize health and longevity.[32] The physiological diet most suitable for humans will also be offered as a science based concept that suggests an ideal food ratio and type based on the typical diet chosen by our closest wild-living great ape relatives, the chimpanzees and bonobos.

By embracing the wisdom of traditional ancestral diets and contemporary nutritional science, we can unravel the secrets of a balanced plate, a culinary masterpiece that not only satisfies the palate but nourishes the body for an extended lifetime of enduring vitality.

BUILDING BLOCKS OF A NUTRIENT-RICH DIET

When studying longevity, the foundational building blocks of our diet assume the role of architects, shaping the contours of our well-being. Dr. Joel Fuhrman, in his illuminating work "Eat to Live," serves as our guide through the labyrinth of nutrient-rich nutrition, emphasizing that the key to optimal health lies not merely in the quantity of calories but, more critically, in the quality of nutrients that our food provides.[33]

---

[31] T. Colin Campbell, Howard Jacobson, "Whole: Rethinking the Science of Nutrition," BenBella Books, 2013.
[32] Joel Fuhrman, "Eat to Live: The Amazing Nutrient-Rich Program for Fast and Sustained Weight Loss," Little, Brown and Company, 2003.
[33] Joel Fuhrman, ibid.

Nutrient Density Unveiled

The concept of nutrient density transcends the conventional understanding of a balanced diet. Dr. Fuhrman contends that nutrient-dense foods, rich in vitamins, minerals, and phytonutrients, form the bedrock of a healthful existence.

As you start to prioritize eating foods with high nutrient density, you can move beyond calorie counting to embrace a culinary journey where each bite becomes full of essential macronutrients, micronutrients and other health-promoting elements.[34]

Dr. Michael Greger, in "How Not to Die," echoes the sentiment by showcasing the transformative potential of plant-based nutrition in preventing and reversing chronic diseases.[35] The amalgamation of scientific research and real-world examples underscores the profound impact of nutrient-dense choices on our health destinies.

The Nutritarian Diet

In his book "Eat to Live", Dr. Fuhrman introduces the Nutritarian approach, advocating for a dietary paradigm where a significant portion of our plate is dedicated to nutrient-rich foods. The fundamental principle of the Nutritarian Diet revolves around the concept that the quantity of nutrients per calorie consumed plays a key role in determining weight and influencing long-term health.

To achieve this, the diet prioritizes nutrient-dense foods, emphasizing whole and minimally processed options while limiting the intake of highly processed ones.

While the Nutritarian Diet doesn't impose strict calorie restrictions, it instead establishes a percentage range of total daily calories that each food group should contribute. These recommendations include:[36]

- **Vegetables (30–60%):** Unlimited consumption is encouraged, with an emphasis on raw veggies constituting at least half of the total vegetable intake daily, excluding potatoes.

---

[34] Joel Fuhrman, ibid.
[35] Michael Greger, Gene Stone, "How Not to Die: Discover the Foods Scientifically Proven to Prevent and Reverse Disease," Flatiron Books, 2015.
[36] Joel Fuhrman, ibid.

- **Fruits (10–40%):** Aim for a minimum of 3–5 servings of fresh fruit daily.
- **Beans and Legumes (10–40%):** Consume at least 1/2 cup (85 grams) daily.
- **Nuts, Seeds, and Avocados (10–40%):** Include at least 1 ounce (28 grams) daily, but moderation is advised for optimal weight loss.
- **Whole Grains and Potatoes (20% maximum):** For weight loss, restrict cooked starches to 1 cup (150–325 grams) daily until reaching the ideal body mass index (BMI).
- **Non-Factory-Farmed Animal Products (less than 10%):** Limit consumption of all animal products, including meat, dairy, eggs, fish, and seafood, as much as possible, and ideally keep this category to less than 8 ounces (225 grams) weekly.
- **Minimally Processed Foods (less than 10%):** This category encompasses tofu, tempeh, and coarsely ground or sprouted whole grain breads and cereals.
- **Sweets, Processed Foods, and Factory-Farmed Meat and Dairy (minimal):** Consume these items rarely or ideally not at all.

Furthermore, the Nutritarian Diet discourages snacking and recommends replacing one meal daily with a vegetable salad featuring a dressing based on nuts or seeds. The diet imposes a limit of less than 1,000 mg of salt intake per day.

Prohibited items include processed foods, refined carbs, oils, sugar, soda, fruit drinks or juices, white flour, and all factory-farmed animal products. To address potential nutrient deficiencies, adherents are advised to take a multivitamin containing B12, iodine, zinc, and vitamin D, along with an algae oil supplement.

The Physiological Dietary Approach

Another science-based approach to finding a natural and maximally nourishing diet for humans is to look at the diet eaten by other creatures who share our physiology and that we may share a common evolutionary ancestor with.

By looking at the physiological dietary model that other great apes living wild naturally consume, it helps provide us with a blueprint for crafting plates that prioritize health and longevity.

Primatologists report that the typical observed dietary ratio of other great apes like the chimpanzees and bonobos who are most closely related to humans genetically consists of 50 percent fruits, 40 percent leafy greens, and 10 percent other largely plant-based foods.

Anthropological evidence suggests that this modern great ape diet is likely to have also been consumed for millions of years by direct human ancestors living in the Pliocene Era.

Maintaining a strategic food distribution of this type helps ensure not only satiety but also an optimal balance of essential nutrients for cellular rejuvenation and overall well-being. Since nature has adapted our closest living cousins to currently consume food in this ratio, and such a diet probably also nourished our direct ancestors, it follows that humans should also thrive on a similar diet since they have a similar digestive system.

Although few present-day humans manage to get close to that ideal dietary ratio in practice, those that do tend to find extraordinary well-being awaiting them. One key factor that may explain why humans do so well on a physiological diet similar to that of other great apes is that they are consuming the food they are best adapted to eat in its most natural raw state.

This means they get more digestive enzymes and the essential C and B vitamins that would be destroyed by cooking. This fact alone argues for leaving one's food as raw and close to nature as possible to maximize its nutritional value.

Real-World Examples of Nutrient-Rich Diets

Traditional diets, such as those observed in the Blue Zones where individuals experience extraordinary longevity, underscore the significance of nutrient-dense eating. The Okinawan diet, with its emphasis on colorful vegetables, sweet potatoes, and legumes, aligns closely with the Nutritarian and physiological diet principles and contributes to the region's exceptional health outcomes.[37]

Dr. T. Colin Campbell's comprehensive research in "The China Study" reinforces the importance of plant-centric nutrition in promoting health and preventing diseases.[38] These examples from diverse cultures and the

---

[37] Bradley J. Willcox, D. Craig Willcox, Makoto Suzuki, "The Okinawa Program: How the World's Longest-Lived People Achieve Everlasting Health," Clarkson Potter, 2001.
[38] T. Colin Campbell, Thomas M. Campbell II, "The China Study: Revised and

scientific community collectively emphasize that the building blocks of a nutrient-rich diet are not confined to specific regions but are universal principles that transcend geographical boundaries.

As you work toward crafting a well-balanced plate, the foundation of nutrient-rich choices becomes the cornerstone. By embracing the Nutritarian philosophy and consuming food type ratios closer to those suitable for our ideal physiological diet shared by our fellow primates, we not only nourish our bodies but unlock the natural transformative potential of food as a catalyst for optimal health and enduring vitality.

EMBRACING FRUITS AND GREENS IN ABUNDANCE

In the vibrant canvas of a balanced plate, the kaleidoscopic hues of fruits and greens emerge as the brushstrokes that paint a portrait of health and vitality.

Dr. Michael Greger, in his comprehensive exploration "How Not to Die," illuminates the transformative power inherent in the abundant consumption of fruits and greens, underscoring their unparalleled benefits for optimal health.[39]

Filling Up With Fruits

Fruits, with their natural sweetness and an array of vital nutrients, stand as ambassadors of health. Dr. Greger navigates through scientific literature, revealing how the consumption of fruits is closely linked to a reduced risk of chronic diseases.

From the antioxidant-rich berries to the vitamin-packed citrus fruits, each bite becomes a delicious investment in longevity. The proposed ratio of 50 percent fruits in the primate dietary pattern aligns with this emphasis, encouraging us to savor the succulence of nature's bounty.

The Importance of Greens

Greens, the verdant superheroes of the plant kingdom, assume a pivotal

---

Expanded Edition," BenBella Books, 2016
[39] Michael Greger, Gene Stone, "How Not to Die: Discover the Foods Scientifically Proven to Prevent and Reverse Disease," Flatiron Books, 2015.

role in crafting a plate that exudes vitality. Dr. Joel Fuhrman extols the virtues of greens in "Eat to Live," portraying them as nutritional powerhouses dense with essential vitamins, minerals, and phytochemicals.[40]

Scientific research underscores the benefits of leafy greens in promoting cardiovascular health, enhancing cognitive function, and mitigating the risks of chronic diseases.[41] The proposed 40 percent allocation to greens in the ideal primate diet further accentuates their significance in the quest for optimal health.

Nutrient-Rich Diversity

The synergy between fruits and greens becomes a symphony of nutrient-rich diversity, where each element complements the other in a harmonious dance of flavors and health benefits.

Traditional diets, such as the Mediterranean diet celebrated for its plant-centric principles, exemplify the fusion of fruits and greens as a culinary tradition associated with longevity. [42] By embracing this synergy, we not only elevate the sensory experience of our meals but also fortify our bodies with the holistic nutrition they crave.

As illustrated by the chosen diet of our fellow primates, the most suitable dietary ratio based on our physiological characteristics involves a strategic allocation of 50 percent fruits and 40 percent greens.

This reflects the intuitive wisdom distilled from nutritional science and following real-world examples like those provided by our fellow great apes the chimpanzees and bonobos who share a very similar digestive physiology to ours.

Aiming for nutrient-rich diversity beckons us to savor the abundance of fruits and greens, not as mere components of a meal but as essential pillars supporting our path towards enduring health.

---

[40] Joel Fuhrman, "Eat to Live: The Amazing Nutrient-Rich Program for Fast and Sustained Weight Loss," Little, Brown and Company, 2003.

[41] Michael Greger, Gene Stone, ibid.

[42] Ramón Estruch, et al., "Primary Prevention of Cardiovascular Disease with a Mediterranean Diet Supplemented with Extra-Virgin Olive Oil or Nuts," *The New England Journal of Medicine*, 2018.

When crafting a balanced plate, the celebration of fruits and greens in abundance emerges as a path to greater well-being, inviting us to embrace the blend of flavors and nutrients that nature generously provides.

INCORPORATING VEGETABLES, WHOLE GRAINS, LEGUMES, NUTS, AND SEEDS

In crafting a well-balanced plate, the strategic combination of vegetables, whole grains, legumes, nuts, and seeds into the remaining 10 percent of our physiological diet (after the 90 percent composed of fruits and greens) becomes a key way to blend flavors, textures, and nutritional richness successfully.

Dr. T. Colin Campbell, in his seminal work "Whole," unfolds the holistic benefits of integrating these diverse elements into our diet, highlighting their roles in promoting health and preventing diseases.[43]

The Verdant Bounty of Vegetables

Vegetables, diverse in color and nutrient content, are the botanical architects of our health. Dr. Campbell's research emphasizes the key role of vegetables in supplying essential vitamins, minerals, and antioxidants.

From cruciferous broccoli, cabbage and cauliflower to carotenoid-rich carrots, each vegetable contributes its unique spectrum of health-promoting compounds.[44]

The physiological dietary approach advocates for a 10 percent allocation to plant-based foods other than fruits and greens, and this more modest portion is where a variety of raw vegetables can contribute added nutrients to a well-rounded plate.

The Satiating Ability of Whole Grains

Whole grains, with their intact bran and germ, embody a nutritional opulence that transcends refined counterparts.

---

[43] T. Colin Campbell, Howard Jacobson, "Whole: Rethinking the Science of Nutrition," BenBella Books, 2013.
[44] T. Colin Campbell, Howard Jacobson, ibid.

Dr. Campbell underscores the benefits of whole grains in maintaining a healthy weight, regulating blood sugar levels, and fortifying the body with essential nutrients.[45]

The inclusion of whole grains in the 10% portion of the ideal 50-40-10 physiological dietary ratio will amplify the satiating power of our plates, ensuring sustained energy and a wholesome nutritional profile.

Legumes: Protein Powerhouses

Legumes, heralded as protein powerhouses, play a pivotal role in crafting a plate rich in essential amino acids. Dr. Michael Greger, in "How Not to Die," explains the myriad benefits of legumes, from their cardiovascular protective effects to their potential in preventing certain cancers. [46]

The 50-40-10 distribution recognizes the significance of legumes, ensuring that our plates are not only delicious but also abundant in plant-based protein.

Including Nuts and Seeds

Nuts and seeds, with their abundance of healthy fats, protein, and micronutrients, add a layer of resilience to our nutritional palate. Dr. Joel Fuhrman, in "Eat to Live," explores their cardiovascular benefits, emphasizing their role in promoting satiety and contributing to overall well-being. [47]

His Nutritarian dietary philosophy would have us integrate nuts and seeds into the 10 percent allocation remaining after fruits and greens have been consumed. This inclusion recognizes the value of these fat-containing and calorie-dense foods as essential components of a balanced and health-promoting diet.

Contemporary Example: The Mediterranean Diet

Traditional diets, such as those found in regions adhering to the Mediterranean lifestyle, epitomize the harmonious integration of vegetables,

---

[45] T. Colin Campbell, Howard Jacobson, ibid.

[46] Michael Greger, Gene Stone, "How Not to Die: Discover the Foods Scientifically Proven to Prevent and Reverse Disease," Flatiron Books, 2015.

[47] Joel Fuhrman, "Eat to Live: The Amazing Nutrient-Rich Program for Fast and Sustained Weight Loss," Little, Brown and Company, 2003.

whole grains, legumes, nuts, and seeds.

The physiologically-ideal 50-40-10 dietary ratio is quite consistent with these long-standing human dietary traditions, encouraging us to approach our plates with a culinary artistry that honors both the wisdom of the past and the nutritional science of the present.[48]

In the kaleidoscope of a balanced plate, the inclusion of vegetables, whole grains, legumes, nuts, and seeds in modest amounts becomes a celebration of nutritional diversity in a longevity and health-promoting diet.

Overall, the physiological dietary approach, with its ideal 50-40-10 ratio, offers a guiding compass for crafting nutritionally-satisfying plates that not only tantalize the taste buds but also nourish the body with the richness it craves for enduring health.

If you would like to see for yourself what a difference consuming a raw food diet consistent with your great ape physiology can make to your life and health, you will find a week's worth of meal plans containing tantalizing raw food dishes in Appendix B based on the 50-40-10 dietary ratio.

---

[48] Ramón Estruch, et al., "Primary Prevention of Cardiovascular Disease with a Mediterranean Diet Supplemented with Extra-Virgin Olive Oil or Nuts," *The New England Journal of Medicine*, 2018.

CHAPTER 3: EXERCISE FOR LIFE

INTRODUCTION

When it comes to enhancing longevity, the symbiotic partnership between a nourishing diet and regular physical activity takes center stage. This chapter serves as a study into the realm of movement and how it impacts health, exploring the boost that cardiovascular and strength training offer for a life brimming with vitality.

As you study the topic of exercise, expect to unearth the secrets to an active and healthy longevity as you explore the science-based benefits of physical fitness and start to discover the profound joy embedded in moving your body.

Embarking on the path to greater longevity involves a commitment to regular exercise, a fundamental tenet emphasized by experts in the field. For example, renowned preventive medicine specialist Dr. David Katz underscores the pivotal role of physical activity in promoting overall health and longevity in his book "Disease-Proof: Slash Your Risk of Heart Disease, Cancer, Diabetes, and More—by 80 Percent." [49]

Scientific literature consistently correlates regular exercise with a reduced risk of chronic diseases, improved cardiovascular health, and enhanced mental well-being.[50] As you step into the world of movement, acknowledge the transformative potential of exercise as a cornerstone for a life marked by enduring health.

Cardiovascular and strength training also emerge as the dynamic duo in

---

[49] David L. Katz, "Disease-Proof: Slash Your Risk of Heart Disease, Cancer, Diabetes, and More—by 80 Percent," Hudson Street Press, 2008.
[50] U.S. Department of Health and Human Services, "Physical Activity Guidelines for Americans," 2nd edition, 2018.

sculpting a robust and resilient physique. In addition to his chapters on diet, Dr. Michael Greger, in "How Not to Die," goes into the science behind exercise and its profound impact on cardiovascular health, immune function, and disease prevention.[51]

Cardiovascular exercises, such as brisk walking, running, or cycling, enhance heart health and boost circulation, while strength training activities, like weightlifting or bodyweight exercises, fortify muscles and bones.[52] The synergy between these two modalities becomes a beacon guiding us toward a holistic approach to physical fitness.

Beyond the realm of physiological benefits, finding joy in physical activity can become an integral aspect of a sustainable exercise routine. Dr. John Ratey, in "Spark: The Revolutionary New Science of Exercise and the Brain," explores the profound impact of exercise on mental well-being, emphasizing its role in reducing stress, improving mood, and enhancing cognitive function.[53]

Whether it's a fun dance class, an inspiring nature walk, or a serene yoga session, the key to good mental health lies in discovering physical activities that resonate with your individual preferences and bring you a deep sense of fulfillment. The pursuit of joy in movement transforms exercise from a mere obligation into a source of lasting pleasure, fostering a lifelong commitment to a physically active lifestyle.

In the pages of the sections that follow, you will learn about the connections between exercise and longevity, as you explore the physiological wonders that unfold when nourishing our bodies with a raw plant-based diet finds its complement in the enjoyment of physical activity. Together, they converge as the twin pillars of a life marked by vibrancy, resilience, and the sheer joy of movement.

MOVING TOWARDS LONGEVITY

When it comes to promoting greater longevity, the rhythm of your steps

[51] Michael Greger, Gene Stone, "How Not to Die: Discover the Foods Scientifically Proven to Prevent and Reverse Disease," Flatiron Books, 2015.
[52] American Council on Exercise (ACE), "Strength Training 101: What You Need to Know," 2021.
[53] John J. Ratey, Eric Hagerman, "Spark: The Revolutionary New Science of Exercise and the Brain," Little, Brown Spark, 2008.

and the cadence of your heartbeats intertwine with the very essence of your existence. The end result is that moving your body more tends to extend your life.

Among the many researchers who have studied this key correlation, Dr. David Katz is a prominent advocate of preventive medicine. He asserts that regular physical activity is not just a choice but a fundamental key to unlocking the doors to enduring health.[54]

Humans Evolved to Move

Our evolutionary history highlights our ancient survival-related needs for movement. It lays the foundation for the intrinsic connection between physical activity and longevity.

Renowned paleoanthropologist Dr. Daniel Lieberman posits that our plant food-gathering ancestors were in almost constant motion, and that this active lifestyle has indelibly shaped the physiological blueprint of the human body.[55]

In the contemporary context, adopting a lifestyle that mirrors this evolutionary legacy becomes very helpful since it helps foster a harmonious alliance between our bodies and our innate need for movement.

The Cellular Basis of Exercise's Benefits

When exploring the microcosm of our cellular composition, exercise emerges as a rejuvenating act.

Cellular biologist Dr. Bruce Lipton has explored the transformative impact of physical activity at the cellular level. In his research, he highlights movement's role in enhancing mitochondrial function, promoting cellular repair, and optimizing metabolic pathways.[56]

These cellular-level interactions become the undercurrent that propels us towards a state of enhanced vitality and longevity.

---

[54] David L. Katz, "Disease-Proof: Slash Your Risk of Heart Disease, Cancer, Diabetes, and More—by 80 Percent," Hudson Street Press, 2008.
[55] Daniel E. Lieberman, "The Story of the Human Body: Evolution, Health, and Disease," Vintage, 2014.
[56] Bruce H. Lipton, "The Biology of Belief: Unleashing the Power of Consciousness, Matter & Miracles," Hay House, 2005.

A Shield Against Chronic Diseases

The scientific consensus on the protective shield that regular exercise constructs against chronic diseases is resounding and offers a very compelling reason to start moving your body now.

Research, such as that presented in the "Physical Activity Guidelines for Americans," establishes the correlation between physical activity and a reduced risk of heart disease, type 2 diabetes, certain cancers, and other serious and chronic adverse health conditions that can definitely shorten your lifespan.[57]

The shield exercise provides can become our armor, fortifying our bodies against the onslaught of ailments that can threaten our good health and longevity.

Beyond the Cardiovascular Benefits

The benefits of exercise extend beyond the cardiovascular realm, permeating into the complex network of our bodily systems.

In his excellent book "How Not to Die," Dr. Michael Greger synthesizes his extensive research to illuminate how physical activity contributes not only to heart health but also to enhanced immune function, improved mental well-being, and a reduced risk of age-related cognitive decline.[58]

This holistic perspective positions exercise as a transformative force that can permeate the fabric of our entire physical and psychological being.

The Synergy with a Physiologically-Appropriate Diet

You should be realizing by now that aligning the health-promoting momentum of movement with the principles of a plant-based physiological diet is a major key to enjoying optimal health.

The ideal 50-40-10 dietary ratio that our fellow great ape cousins naturally gravitate toward when living in the wild also serves as a complementary lifestyle addition that amplifies the benefits derived from physical

[57] U.S. Department of Health and Human Services, "Physical Activity Guidelines for Americans," 2nd edition, 2018.
[58] Michael Greger, Gene Stone, "How Not to Die: Discover the Foods Scientifically Proven to Prevent and Reverse Disease," Flatiron Books, 2015.

movement in a longevity-focused lifestyle.

The synergy between consuming a suitable and nourishing diet for your species and regular exercise becomes the linchpin in the pursuit of a life not just marked by the passage of years but by the enduring vibrancy of each one.

As you step further into the study of enhancing longevity, remain guided by the dietary insights of evolutionary biology and join in the harmonious dance of the cellular benefits you derive from moving regularly.

Remember, engaging in regular physical activity helps unlock the doors to enduring health, taking you further along the path towards a bright horizon where every step becomes a testament to the artistry of a life lived with purpose and good health.

CARDIOVASCULAR AND STRENGTH TRAINING

When examining the mechanics of an effective exercise regimen, the spotlight inevitably falls on the symbiotic relationship between cardiovascular and strength training.

Grounded in scientific rigor, this section explains the physiological details and health implications of integrating these two modalities into a comprehensive fitness routine.

Cardiovascular Training for Better Cardiovascular Health

Cardiovascular exercises, typified by activities such as running, cycling, and swimming, constitute the bedrock of aerobic fitness. Referencing comprehensive studies in his book "How Not to Die," Dr. Michael Greger delineates the cardiovascular benefits of regular aerobic training.

Improved cardiac output, enhanced blood vessel function, and lowered blood pressure are among the positive outcomes he has documented, all contributing to a reduced risk of cardiovascular diseases.[59]

Notably, data from the American Heart Association reinforces the positive correlation between sustained cardiovascular activity and a decreased

---

[59] Michael Greger, Gene Stone, "How Not to Die: Discover the Foods Scientifically Proven to Prevent and Reverse Disease," Flatiron Books, 2015.

incidence of heart-related ailments.[60]

Strength Training to Build Muscular Resilience

Strength training, often involving resistance exercises like weightlifting, emerges as a pivotal component in fortifying the musculoskeletal system. Dr. Miriam Nelson's research, particularly in "Strong Women Stay Young," underscores the role of strength training in promoting lean muscle mass, bone density, and metabolic efficiency.[61]

The scientific consensus, as acknowledged by institutions like the American College of Sports Medicine (ACSM), solidifies the importance of resistance training in preventing age-related muscle loss and fostering overall musculoskeletal health.[62]

Synergy of Cardiovascular and Strength Training

The amalgamation of cardiovascular and strength training ushers in a holistic approach to fitness. ACE's guidelines highlight the complementary nature of these modalities where cardiovascular exercises enhance endurance, promote calorie expenditure, and improve overall cardiovascular health.

Furthermore, strength training bolsters muscular strength, preserves bone density, and augments metabolic function.[63] This synergy is underscored by research published in the Journal of Strength and Conditioning Research, emphasizing the combined benefits of simultaneous cardiovascular and resistance training.[64]

Cognitive and Physiological Benefits of Exercise

---

[60] American Heart Association, "Physical Activity and Cardiovascular Health," 2021.

[61] Miriam E. Nelson, "Strong Women Stay Young: Revised Edition," Bantam, 2019.

[62] American College of Sports Medicine (ACSM), "ACSM Position Stand on Progression Models in Resistance Training for Healthy Adults," *Medicine & Science in Sports & Exercise*, 2009.

[63] American Council on Exercise (ACE), "Cardiovascular Exercise vs. Resistance Training," 2021.

[64] M. J. Peterson, et al., "Resistance Exercise for Muscular Strength in Older Adults: A Meta-Analysis," *Ageing Research Reviews*, 2011.

Beyond the apparent physical gains, exercise—both cardiovascular and strength training—acts as a catalyst for cognitive and physiological well-being. Dr. John Ratey's exploration in "Spark: The Revolutionary New Science of Exercise and the Brain" delves into the neurotrophic factors released during strength training, fostering the growth and preservation of brain cells.[65]

Scientific understanding, exemplified by studies in the Journal of Applied Physiology, reinforces the cognitive benefits derived from both modalities of exercise.[66]

Overall, a robust exercise regimen encompasses the symbiotic interplay of cardiovascular and strength training. The scientific consensus aligns with the pragmatic integration of these modalities, promoting not only physiological health but also cognitive well-being.

As you explore exercise physiology further, you will discover a roadmap to enduring health, where the combination of cardiovascular and strength training resonates with the principles of a raw plant-based physiological diet, setting the stage for optimal well-being and graceful aging.

ENJOYING PHYSICAL ACTIVITY

When examining the importance of physical activity, taking a closer look at the psychological dimensions becomes imperative. This section explores the cognitive intricacies, behavioral paradigms, and neuroscientific underpinnings that collectively contribute to the pursuit of joy within the realm of exercise.

The Psychological Dynamics of Exercise

Understanding the psychology of exercise entails a study of cognitive processes and their profound impact on behavior. Dr. Albert Bandura's Social Cognitive Theory provides a foundational framework, emphasizing the role of self-efficacy—the belief in one's capability to execute a specific behavior—in shaping exercise habits. [67]

---

[65] John J. Ratey, Eric Hagerman, "Spark: The Revolutionary New Science of Exercise and the Brain," Little, Brown Spark, 2008.
[66] M. Yoon, et al., "Effects of resistance exercise on cognitive function," *Journal of Strength and Conditioning Research*, 2007.
[67] Albert Bandura, "Social Foundations of Thought and Action: A Social Cognitive

The cognitive appraisal of personal competence becomes a pivotal determinant in the initiation, maintenance, and adherence to regular exercise routines. As individuals develop a robust sense of self-efficacy through successful experiences and positive feedback loops, the likelihood of engaging in and persisting with physical activity is significantly heightened.

Intrinsic vs. Extrinsic Motivation

Motivational forces driving exercise behavior can be categorized into intrinsic and extrinsic factors, a behavioral paradigm elucidated by Deci and Ryan's Self-Determination Theory.[68]

Intrinsic motivation, characterized by engaging in activities for inherent satisfaction and personal enjoyment, emerges as a potent catalyst for sustaining long-term adherence to exercise routines. In contrast, extrinsic motivation, driven by external rewards or avoidance of punishment, tends to be less sustainable over time.

Fostering intrinsic motivation involves aligning physical activities with personal values, interests, and a sense of autonomy, establishing a foundation where the inherent joy derived from the exercise itself becomes a sustainable driver for engagement.

The Role of Dopamine

At the neuroscientific level, the pursuit of joy in physical activity is closely linked to the release of dopamine, a neurotransmitter associated with pleasure and reward.

Exercise induces the activation of dopamine pathways in the brain's reward centers, creating a neurobiological response that reinforces positive associations with physical activity.[69]

This neurochemical interplay not only enhances the immediate pleasure derived from exercise but also contributes to the formation of long-term

---

Theory," Prentice-Hall, 1986.
[68] Edward L. Deci, Richard M. Ryan, "Intrinsic Motivation and Self-Determination in Human Behavior," Plenum Press, 1985.
[69] Wendy A. Suzuki, "Healthy Brain, Happy Life: A Personal Program to Activate Your Brain and Do Everything Better," Dey Street Books, 2015.

positive attitudes toward physical activity.

As individuals experience the neurochemical rewards of exercise, they are more likely to seek out and sustain activities that bring them joy, establishing a reinforcing loop that supports ongoing engagement.

Exercise as a Stress Regulator

The stress-regulating effects of exercise offer a profound perspective on the mental health benefits inherent in physical activity. Cortisol, a hormone associated with the body's stress response, exhibits dynamic fluctuations in response to exercise.

Studies, such as those published in the Journal of Behavioral Medicine, underscore the role of exercise in modulating cortisol levels and mitigating the impact of chronic stressors.[70] The interplay between cortisol regulation and psychological well-being positions exercise as a potent tool for stress management.

Engaging in regular physical activity not only provides a physiological outlet for the body's stress response but also cultivates a psychological resilience that contributes to overall mental well-being.

Behavioral Activation and Mental Health

Behavioral activation, grounded in behavioral psychology, offers a clinical lens through which the positive impact of enjoyable activities, including exercise, on mental health is examined.[71]

Dr. Martin Seligman's PERMA model further underscores the multifaceted nature of mental well-being, encompassing positive emotion, engagement, relationships, meaning, and accomplishment.[72]

Integrating exercise into daily life becomes a practical strategy for enhancing mental health, as the positive emotions and sense of accomplishment derived from physical activity contribute to a flourishing psychological state.

---

[70] S. E. Salmon, L. L. Kegeles, "The Role of Coping in Exercise Participation for Persons with Previous Exercise Experience," *Journal of Behavioral Medicine*, 1995.

[71] C. Martell, M. Dimidjian, R. Herman-Dunn, "Behavioral Activation for Depression: A Clinician's Guide," Guilford Press, 2010.

[72] Martin E. P. Seligman, "Flourish: A Visionary New Understanding of Happiness and Well-being," Free Press, 2011.

Personalization and Enjoyment Over the Long-Term

The sustained enjoyment of physical activity hinges on the personalization of exercise routines. Tailoring activities to individual preferences, interests, and capabilities fosters a sense of autonomy and increases the likelihood of continued engagement. [73]

This individualized approach acknowledges that the pursuit of joy in exercise is inherently subjective and requires a nuanced understanding of personal preferences.

Whether it's exploring various forms of exercise, participating in group activities, or embracing outdoor pursuits, the key lies in aligning physical activity with what brings individuals genuine enjoyment.

Incorporating Fun into Your Exercise Program

A real-world application of the principles discussed in this section could involve translating the theoretical constructs of joy in exercise into practical strategies for sustained engagement.

Community-based fitness classes, team sports, and group activities exemplify how the social and enjoyable aspects of physical activity can be leveraged to enhance adherence.

Scientifically grounded interventions, as outlined in the Journal of Consulting and Clinical Psychology, emphasize the integration of enjoyable activities as a means to enhance exercise adherence.[74]

By aligning physical activity with personal preferences and creating a supportive social environment, individuals can navigate the complexities of real-world commitments while finding joy in their exercise routines.

In conclusion, the pursuit of joy in physical activity transcends a mere desire for pleasure—it is a multifaceted interplay of cognitive, behavioral, and neurobiological processes.

---

[73] American College of Sports Medicine (ACSM), "Quantity and Quality of Exercise for Developing and Maintaining Cardiorespiratory, Musculoskeletal, and Neuromotor Fitness in Apparently Healthy Adults: Guidance for Prescribing Exercise," *Medicine & Science in Sports & Exercise*, 2011.

[74] M. G. Perri, et al., "Improving the maintenance of weight lost in behavioral treatment of obesity," *Journal of Consulting and Clinical Psychology*, 1984.

As individuals strive to embed joy into their exercise habits, the conscious integration of these psychological dimensions becomes instrumental in fostering a sustainable and rewarding relationship with physical activity.

CHAPTER 4: QUALITY SLEEP MATTERS

INTRODUCTION

When looking to increase longevity, the role of quality sleep emerges as an important factor in supporting general health and well-being. This chapter explores the detailed mechanisms governing a restful night, unveils the science behind cultivating healthy sleep habits, and explores the profound link between sleep and longevity.

Adequate and quality sleep, as expounded by Dr. Matthew Walker in "Why We Sleep," is an often-underestimated pillar of health. Walker's seminal work illustrates the critical role sleep plays in memory consolidation, immune function, and cellular repair, offering profound insights into how our nightly rest contributes to overall longevity.[75]

The pursuit of a restful night's sleep involves unraveling the secrets of sleep architecture and the neurochemicals orchestrating this nightly event. Walker's research provides a comprehensive exploration of sleep cycles, from the alternating stages of non-REM and REM sleep to the critical role of circadian rhythms. Understanding the nuances of these sleep phases unveils the significance of each in physiological restoration, memory consolidation, and overall cognitive function.

Further delving into the neurobiology, Dr. Robert Stickgold's research underscores the role of sleep in synaptic plasticity—the strengthening and consolidation of neural connections essential for learning and memory. [76]As we explore the mechanics of a restful night, it becomes evident that quality sleep is not a passive state but an active and essential process for physical and cognitive rejuvenation.

The path to quality sleep is paved with the establishment of healthy sleep habits, grounded in evidence-based practices. Sleep hygiene principles, as advocated by the American Academy of Sleep Medicine (AASM), offer

---

[75] Matthew Walker, "Why We Sleep: Unlocking the Power of Sleep and Dreams," Scribner, 2017.
[76] Robert Stickgold, "Sleep-dependent memory consolidation," *Nature*, 2005.

actionable strategies for optimizing sleep quality.[77] These encompass maintaining a consistent sleep schedule, creating a conducive sleep environment, and fostering bedtime routines that signal the body's transition into rest.

Dr. Michael Grandner's research further underscores the impact of lifestyle factors on sleep, emphasizing the role of physical activity, nutrition, and stress management in shaping sleep quality.[78] By aligning daily habits with circadian rhythms and adopting personalized sleep hygiene practices, individuals can pave the way for consistent and restorative sleep.

The profound link between sleep and longevity extends beyond the realms of physical and cognitive restoration. Epidemiological studies, including those referenced in the "Sleep Duration and Quality: Impact on Lifestyle Behaviors and Cardiometabolic Health" report, illuminate the associations between inadequate sleep and an increased risk of chronic diseases.[79] Cardiovascular health, metabolic function, and immune resilience are closely intertwined with the quantity and quality of sleep one receives.

Dr. Valter Longo's exploration of the molecular underpinnings in "The Longevity Diet" sheds light on how sleep influences cellular repair and regeneration.[80] Sleep deprivation not only disrupts hormonal balance, impacting appetite and metabolism but also compromises the body's ability to undergo autophagy—a cellular cleanup process that is very conducive to longevity.

When exploring the relationship between sleep quality and longevity, it becomes evident that prioritizing a healthy sleep pattern is a cornerstone for enhancing not only the duration of life but the vibrancy and vitality within the years lived.

---

[77] American Academy of Sleep Medicine (AASM), "Sleep Hygiene," 2020.

[78] Michael A. Grandner, et al., "Sleep: Important Considerations for the Prevention of Cardiovascular Disease," *Current Opinion in Cardiology*, 2016.

[79] National Sleep Foundation, "Sleep Duration and Quality: Impact on Lifestyle Behaviors and Cardiometabolic Health," 2021.

[80] Valter Longo, "The Longevity Diet: Discover the New Science Behind Stem Cell Activation and Regeneration to Slow Aging, Fight Disease, and Optimize Weight," Avery, 2018.

UNLOCKING THE SECRETS OF A RESTFUL NIGHT

Within sleep architecture, the secrets of a restful night lie deeply involved with a person's neurobiology and circadian rhythms.

As we explore the scientific basis of sleep cycles, the alternating stages of non-REM (Rapid Eye Movement) and REM sleep unveil a choreographed pattern of physiological processes.

Understanding Sleep Cycles and Restoration

Dr. Matthew Walker's research, encapsulated in "Why We Sleep," unravels the profound significance of sleep cycles. Non-REM sleep, divided into four stages, initiates the process of restoration.

Stages 1 and 2 mark the transition from wakefulness to deeper sleep, with the brain undergoing oscillatory patterns conducive to memory consolidation.[81] Stages 3 and 4 involve slow-wave sleep (SWS), characterized by synchronized neuronal activity that is essential for physical rejuvenation and immune function.[82]

Interwoven with these non-REM stages is the enigmatic REM sleep—a period marked by vivid dreaming and heightened brain activity. Dr. Rosalind Cartwright's seminal work dissects the role of REM sleep in emotional processing and cognitive integration, emphasizing its contribution to mental resilience and well-being.[83]

Circadian Rhythm Timing Matters

Beyond the intricacies of sleep stages, the circadian rhythm orchestrates the optimal timing of these cycles. Dr. Joseph Takahashi's groundbreaking research on the molecular mechanisms of circadian clocks elucidates how these internal timekeepers synchronize with external cues, regulating the sleep-wake cycle. [84]

---

[81] Matthew Walker, "Why We Sleep: Unlocking the Power of Sleep and Dreams," Scribner, 2017.

[82] M. P. Walker, "The Role of Sleep in Cognition and Emotion," *Annals of the New York Academy of Sciences*, 2009.

[83] Rosalind D. Cartwright, "The Twenty-Four Hour Mind: The Role of Sleep and Dreaming in Our Emotional Lives," Oxford University Press, 2010.

[84] Joseph S. Takahashi, "Molecular Architecture of the Circadian Clock in

Melatonin, a hormone regulated by the circadian clock, plays a pivotal role in signaling the onset of sleep, as exemplified by studies referenced in the Journal of Pineal Research.[85]

To unlock the secrets of a restful night, aligning sleep with the natural ebb and flow of circadian rhythms becomes paramount. This synchronization optimizes the efficiency of sleep cycles, fostering both physical and cognitive restoration.

Sleep-Inducing Neurochemicals

The neurochemical ballet underlying a restful night involves the orchestrated release of neurotransmitters and neuromodulators. Adenosine, a key player in promoting sleep, accumulates in the brain throughout wakefulness. Dr. Robert McCarley's research sheds light on adenosine's role in initiating sleep by inhibiting wake-promoting neurons.[86]

Concurrently, the delicate balance of serotonin, dopamine, and gamma-aminobutyric acid (GABA) influences the transitions between wakefulness and sleep. Dr. Jean-Pierre Changeux's exploration of the molecular mechanisms regulating these neurotransmitters unravels their pivotal roles in the modulation of sleep-wake states.[87]

As we dissect the neurochemical underpinnings, it becomes evident that a restful night hinges on the synchronized interplay of these molecules, orchestrating the transition from wakefulness to the realms of non-REM and REM sleep.

In sum, unlocking the secrets of a restful night involves a nuanced understanding of sleep cycles, circadian rhythms, and the complex neurochemistry that orchestrates the shift from wakefulness to the rejuvenating realms of sleep.

Mammals," *Science*, 2017.

[85] C. Cajochen, et al., "High Sensitivity of Human Melatonin, Alertness, Thermoregulation, and Heart Rate to Short Wavelength Light," *The Journal of Clinical Endocrinology & Metabolism*, 2005.

[86] Robert W. McCarley, "Neurobiology of REM and NREM Sleep," *Sleep Medicine*, 2007.

[87] Jean-Pierre Changeux, "Neuronal Man: The Biology of Mind," Princeton University Press, 1997

As you navigate the complexities of this nocturnal process, the keys to quality sleep can be found in the scientific revelations that underpin a profound and restorative night's rest.

CREATING HEALTHY SLEEP HABITS

The pursuit of quality sleep transcends the passive act of lying down—it involves the deliberate cultivation of healthy sleep habits. Grounded in evidence-based practices, these habits form the linchpin for optimizing sleep quality and fostering a restorative nocturnal experience.

Sleep Hygiene Principles for Optimal Rest

Sleep hygiene, as delineated by the American Academy of Sleep Medicine (AASM), encapsulates a set of principles instrumental in shaping healthy sleep habits.[88] Maintaining a consistent sleep schedule, even on weekends, aligns with the body's circadian rhythm, optimizing the synchronization of sleep-wake cycles.

This consistency reinforces the internal biological clock, enhancing the efficiency of sleep stages, as corroborated by research published in the journal *Sleep*. [89]

Creating a sleep-conducive environment involves optimizing ambient conditions, such as temperature, light, and noise. Dr. Chris Idzikowski's work emphasizes the role of a cool and dark bedroom in promoting both sleep onset and continuity.[90]

Eliminating extraneous noise through soundproofing measures contributes to uninterrupted sleep, supporting the delicate orchestration of sleep cycles.

How Bedtime Rituals Cue Sleep Induction

Establishing bedtime rituals serves as a behavioral cue signaling the body's

---

[88] American Academy of Sleep Medicine (AASM), "Sleep Hygiene," 2020.

[89] Orfeu M. Buxton, et al., "Adverse Metabolic Consequences in Humans of Prolonged Sleep Restriction Combined with Circadian Disruption," *Science Translational Medicine*, 2012.

[90] Chris Idzikowski, "Sound Asleep: The Expert Guide to Sleeping Well," Kyle Books, 2015.

transition into the realm of sleep. Dr. Michael Grandner's exploration of lifestyle factors influencing sleep underscores the efficacy of consistent pre-sleep routines in promoting relaxation and lowering arousal levels. [91]

Whether through activities like reading, gentle stretching, or mindfulness practices, these rituals create a psychological signal, priming the mind and body for the impending shift into slumber.

Cognitive-Behavioral Strategies for Changing Sleep Patterns

Cognitive-behavioral strategies, rooted in principles of cognitive therapy, play a pivotal role in mitigating sleep disorders and enhancing sleep quality.

Dr. Jack Edinger's research highlights the efficacy of cognitive restructuring—addressing and modifying maladaptive thoughts and beliefs about sleep—in improving overall sleep patterns.[92]

By reshaping perceptions and attitudes towards sleep, individuals can break the cycle of anxiety and promote a more positive relationship with bedtime.

Lifestyle Impact on Sleep Patterns

The impact of lifestyle factors on sleep quality extends beyond the confines of the bedroom. Dr. Michael Irwin's investigation into the reciprocal relationship between physical activity and sleep underscores the bidirectional influence of exercise on sleep quality.[93]

Engaging in regular physical activity not only promotes physical well-being but also contributes to the regulation of circadian rhythms, enhancing the propensity for restful sleep.

Managing stress, a potent disruptor of sleep, emerges as a cornerstone in the pursuit of healthy sleep habits. Mindfulness-based interventions, as outlined by Dr. Jason Ong's research, showcase the efficacy of mindfulness

---

[91] Michael A. Grandner, et al., "A behavioral sleep medicine perspective on insomnia treatment in patients with psychiatric comorbidities," *Behavioral Sleep Medicine*, 2008.

[92] Jack D. Edinger, "Cognitive-Behavioral Therapy for the Treatment of Insomnia," *Chest*, 2009.

[93] Michael R. Irwin, et al., "Improving Sleep Quality in Older Adults with Moderate Sleep Complaints: A Randomized Controlled Trial of Tai Chi Chih," *Sleep*, 2008.

techniques in reducing pre-sleep arousal and fostering a calm mental state conducive to sleep.[94]

Chronobiology Suggests Aligning Habits with Circadian Rhythms

The principles of chronobiology advocate for aligning daily habits with the body's natural circadian rhythms. Dr. Till Roenneberg's work emphasizes the importance of chronotype awareness—understanding one's individual predisposition for morning or evening preference. [95]

Aligning daily activities, including meals and exercise, with one's chronotype optimizes the synchronization of physiological processes, including the sleep-wake cycle.

In conclusion, the creation of healthy sleep habits transcends arbitrary routines—it involves a strategic alignment with the body's intrinsic biological rhythms and the deliberate adoption of evidence-based practices.

As individuals navigate the nuances of sleep hygiene, bedtime rituals, cognitive-behavioral strategies, and lifestyle adjustments, they fortify the foundation for quality sleep—a cornerstone for enhanced health and longevity.

THE LINK BETWEEN SLEEP AND LONGEVITY

The close relationship between sleep and longevity emphasizes the profound influence of sleep quality and duration on overall health and life expectancy.

As the scientific exploration deepens, the evidence underscores the pivotal role of sleep in shaping the trajectory of various physiological processes, ultimately impacting the quantity and quality of one's lifespan.

Nocturnal Patterns and Cardiovascular Health

Cardiovascular health stands as a sentinel example of the complex interplay

---

[94] Jason C. Ong, et al., "A Mindfulness-Based Approach to the Treatment of Insomnia," *Journal of Clinical Psychology*, 2009.

[95] Till Roenneberg, "Internal Time: Chronotypes, Social Jet Lag, and Why You're So Tired," Harvard University Press, 2012.

between sleep and longevity. Dr. Susan Redline's extensive research, as highlighted in the *European Heart Journal*, reveals the close association between insufficient sleep and an elevated risk of cardiovascular diseases.[96]

Chronic sleep deprivation disrupts the delicate balance of autonomic nervous system function, leading to heightened sympathetic activity and increased blood pressure, factors strongly linked to the development of cardiovascular pathologies.

Moreover, the phenomenon of sleep-disordered breathing, exemplified by conditions like sleep apnea, serves as a compelling illustration of your nocturnal experience's impact on cardiovascular health.

Dr. Virend Somers' research elucidates the bidirectional relationship between sleep apnea and cardiovascular morbidity, where untreated sleep apnea not only contributes to the progression of cardiovascular diseases but also serves as an independent risk factor for adverse cardiovascular events.[97]

Nocturnal Metabolic Hormones

The orchestration of metabolic harmony unfolds during the nocturnal hours, with the phenomenon of sleep regulating hormonal balance and various metabolic processes.

Dr. Eve Van Cauter's seminal work on sleep and hormonal regulation delineates the influence of sleep duration on key hormones, such as leptin and ghrelin, that are involved in appetite regulation.[98]

Insufficient sleep disrupts this delicate equilibrium, leading to alterations in appetite, increased caloric intake, and subsequent metabolic dysregulation— an ominous precursor to conditions like obesity and type 2 diabetes especially if a plant-based diet is not being strictly followed.

---

[96] Susan Redline, et al., "Sleep duration and cardiovascular risk: the impact of averaging long-term sleep patterns," *European Heart Journal*, 2018.

[97] Virend K. Somers, et al., "Sleep apnea and cardiovascular disease: An American Heart Association/American College of Cardiology Foundation Scientific Statement from the American Heart Association Council for High Blood Pressure Research Professional Education Committee, Council on Clinical Cardiology, Stroke Council, and Council on Cardiovascular Nursing. In collaboration with the National Heart, Lung, and Blood Institute National Center on Sleep Disorders Research (National Institutes of Health)," *Circulation*, 2008.

[98] Eve Van Cauter, et al., "The Impact of Sleep Deprivation on Hormones and Metabolism," *Medscape Neurology*, 2005.

In the study of metabolic health, sleep thus emerges as a critical determinant of insulin sensitivity. Dr. Josiane Broussard's research, as published in *Diabetes Care*, unveils the bidirectional relationship between sleep duration and insulin sensitivity, emphasizing the vital role of sleep in maintaining metabolic homeostasis.[99]

Disruptions in this delicate balance contribute to the development of insulin resistance—a pivotal factor in the pathogenesis of metabolic disorders with far-reaching implications for longevity.

Immunological Resilience Boosted by Good Sleep Patterns

The link between sleep and longevity extends its influence to the immune system, where the nocturnal hours serve as a critical period for immunological resilience. Dr. Michael Irwin's exploration of sleep and immune function, as presented in *Nature Reviews Immunology*, accentuates the bidirectional relationship between sleep quality and immune responses.[100]

Insufficient or disrupted sleep compromises immune surveillance, increasing susceptibility to infections and impairing the body's ability to mount effective immune defenses.

Chronic sleep deprivation, as investigated by Dr. Nathaniel Watson and colleagues, culminates in a pro-inflammatory internal environment, fostering a chronic state of low-grade inflammation—a phenomenon closely linked to the aging process and age-related diseases.[101]

The balance between pro-inflammatory and anti-inflammatory processes, regulated in part by the quality and duration of sleep, emerges as a key determinant in shaping the trajectory of immunological resilience and overall longevity.

Good Sleep Patterns Protect Against Cognitive Decline

The protective power of sleep extends to neurological integrity, safeguarding against cognitive decline and neurodegenerative disorders.

---

[99] Josiane L. Broussard, et al., "Impaired insulin signaling in human adipocytes after experimental sleep restriction: a randomized, crossover study," *Diabetes Care*, 2012.
[100] Michael R. Irwin, et al., "Sleep and Immune Function," *Nature Reviews Immunology*, 2019.
[101] Nathaniel F. Watson, et al., "Cytokines and Sleep," *Sleep Medicine Clinics*, 2007.

Dr. Maiken Nedergaard's research on the glymphatic system—a waste clearance system active during sleep—reveals how sleep facilitates the removal of neurotoxic byproducts, including beta-amyloid, implicated in the pathogenesis of Alzheimer's disease.[102]

Insufficient sleep disrupts this vital waste clearance mechanism, contributing to the accumulation of neurotoxic substances and accelerating cognitive decline.

Furthermore, the link between sleep and longevity manifests prominently in the association between sleep disorders, such as insomnia, and an increased risk of neurodegenerative conditions.

Dr. Jeffrey Iliff's investigations underscore the bidirectional relationship between sleep quality and the risk of neurodegenerative disorders, illuminating the potential role of sleep interventions in mitigating cognitive decline.[103]

Aligning Sleep with Circadian Rhythms

The chronobiological synchrony between sleep and circadian rhythms emerges as a final factor in the link between sleep and longevity. Dr. Till Roenneberg's research emphasizes the importance of chronotype alignment with societal schedules, advocating for the synchronization of sleep-wake cycles with the intrinsic biological clock.[104]

Disruptions in this synchrony, as seen in shift work or irregular sleep patterns, not only compromise the quality of sleep but also contribute to the dysregulation of various physiological processes, potentially impacting overall longevity.

In essence, the link between sleep and longevity is a multifaceted phenomenon involving cardiovascular health, metabolic harmony, immunological resilience, neurological integrity, and chronobiological synchrony.

[102] Maiken Nedergaard, "Brain Drain," *Scientific American*, 2014.

[103] Jeffrey J. Iliff, et al., "A Paravascular Pathway Facilitates CSF Flow Through the Brain Parenchyma and the Clearance of Interstitial Solutes, Including Amyloid β," *Science Translational Medicine*, 2012.

[104] Till Roenneberg, "Internal Time: Chronotypes, Social Jet Lag, and Why You're So Tired," Harvard University Press, 2012.

As individuals navigate the complexities of modern lifestyles, the recognition of sleep as a potent determinant of longevity underscores the importance of cultivating healthy sleep habits and prioritizing the quality and duration of nightly rest.

51

CHAPTER 5: STRESS MANAGEMENT TECHNIQUES

INTRODUCTION

When studying factors that influence health and longevity, stress management emerges as a pivotal domain, wielding profound implications for both physiological well-being and the pursuit of a long and healthy life. This chapter navigates the nuanced terrain of stress, unraveling its impact on health and delving into evidence-based strategies for its effective mitigation.

The exploration begins with an in-depth examination of the multifaceted impact of stress on health. Dr. Robert Sapolsky's extensive research, as presented in "Why Zebras Don't Get Ulcers," illuminates the physiological cascade triggered by stress, encompassing the release of stress hormones such as cortisol and the activation of the sympathetic nervous system.[105] Chronic exposure to these stress mediators has been implicated in a spectrum of health issues, ranging from cardiovascular diseases to compromised immune function.

The detailed interplay between stress and the immune system stands as a focal point in understanding the broader health ramifications. Dr. Sheldon Cohen's investigations, including studies cited in the "Psychological Stress and Susceptibility to the Common Cold" report, accentuate the immunosuppressive effects of chronic stress, increasing vulnerability to infections.[106]

In addition, stress-induced inflammation, elucidated by research conducted by Dr. George Slavich, contributes to the pathogenesis of numerous chronic conditions, further underscoring the necessity of effective stress management strategies.[107]

---

[105] Robert M. Sapolsky, "Why Zebras Don't Get Ulcers: The Acclaimed Guide to Stress, Stress-Related Diseases, and Coping," Holt Paperbacks, 2004.
[106] Sheldon Cohen, et al., "Psychological Stress and Susceptibility to the Common Cold," *The New England Journal of Medicine*, 1991.
[107] George M. Slavich, "Psychoneuroimmunology of Stress and Mental Health,"

In the arsenal of stress management techniques, mindfulness and meditation emerge as potent tools for cultivating mental resilience and mitigating the physiological toll of stress. Dr. Jon Kabat-Zinn's groundbreaking work in "Full Catastrophe Living" introduces the concept of mindfulness-based stress reduction (MBSR), emphasizing the cultivation of present-moment awareness to alleviate stress and enhance overall well-being.[108]

Scientific investigations into the neurobiological effects of mindfulness and meditation, such as those explored by Dr. Sara Lazar, underscore the structural changes in the brain associated with regular practice.[109] These changes encompass alterations in the amygdala—the brain region central to stress responses—and improvements in prefrontal cortex function, fostering enhanced emotional regulation and resilience in the face of stressors.

The integration of mindfulness into stress management extends beyond mere relaxation techniques—it encapsulates a holistic approach encompassing awareness of bodily sensations, thoughts, and emotions. Dr. Elizabeth Blackburn's research on telomeres—the protective caps at the end of chromosomes—illuminates the potential role of mindfulness in mitigating cellular aging, offering a tangible link between stress reduction and longevity.[110]

The pursuit of a long and healthy life requires the cultivation of resilience—an individual's capacity to adapt positively to stressors and bounce back from adversity. Dr. Ann Masten's research in "Ordinary Magic: Resilience in Development" provides insights into the psychological factors contributing to resilience, emphasizing the importance of fostering a sense of purpose, positive social connections, and adaptive coping strategies.[111]

Psychiatry Clinics of North America, 2019.

[108] Jon Kabat-Zinn, "Full Catastrophe Living: Using the Wisdom of Your Body and Mind to Face Stress, Pain, and Illness," Bantam, 1990.

[109] Sara W. Lazar, et al., "The underlying anatomical correlates of long-term meditation: Larger hippocampal and frontal volumes of gray matter," *NeuroImage*, 2005.

[110] Elizabeth H. Blackburn and Elissa S. Epel, "The Telomere Effect: A Revolutionary Approach to Living Younger, Healthier, Longer," Grand Central Publishing, 2017.

[111] Ann S. Masten, "Ordinary Magic: Resilience in Development," *Guilford Press*, 2014.

The concept of post-traumatic growth, as explored by Dr. Richard Tedeschi and Dr. Lawrence Calhoun, further accentuates the transformative potential inherent in adversity. Instead of merely bouncing back, individuals can undergo positive psychological shifts, leveraging challenges as catalysts for personal growth and enhanced well-being.[112]

In summary, this chapter focuses on stress, unraveling its adverse impacts on human health and introducing evidence-based strategies for its effective management.
From the physiological responses triggered by stress to the transformative potential of mindfulness and the cultivation of resilience, each section of this chapter serves as a compass in guiding individuals away from stress and towards the calming holistic approach required for a long and healthy life.

UNDERSTANDING THE IMPACT OF STRESS ON HEALTH

The complex interaction between stress and health unfolds as a complex physiological cascade, manifesting in a spectrum of outcomes that extend beyond transient psychological discomfort.

A synthesis of empirical research elucidates the multifaceted impact of stress on the human body, delving into hormonal responses, immune modulation, and the potential links to various health disorders.

Stress Hormones and the Neuroendocrine Response

At the core of the stress response lays the complex interplay of hormones, particularly cortisol, orchestrated by the hypothalamic-pituitary-adrenal (HPA) axis. The seminal work of Dr. Bruce McEwen, as encapsulated in "The End of Stress as We Know It," outlines how chronic stress can dysregulate the HPA axis, leading to sustained elevations in cortisol levels.[113]

Prolonged exposure to elevated cortisol is associated with adverse health outcomes, including impaired glucose metabolism, abdominal obesity, and compromised immune function.[114]

---

[112] Richard G. Tedeschi and Lawrence G. Calhoun, "Posttraumatic Growth: Conceptual Foundations and Empirical Evidence," *Psychological Inquiry*, 2004.

[113] Bruce S. McEwen, "The End of Stress as We Know It," Joseph Henry Press, 2002.

[114] Robert M. Sapolsky, "Why Zebras Don't Get Ulcers: The Acclaimed Guide to Stress, Stress-Related Diseases, and Coping," Holt Paperbacks, 2004.

Moreover, the physiological response to stress extends beyond cortisol, involving the release of catecholamines such as epinephrine and norepinephrine.

Dr. Robert Sapolsky's research underscores how these catecholamines contribute to the "fight or flight" response, mobilizing energy resources and modulating cardiovascular function in the face of acute stressors.[115]

Inflammatory Pathways: Stress and Immune Function

The intimate relationship between stress and the immune system unfolds through the modulation of inflammatory pathways. Chronic stress is associated with a proinflammatory state, as highlighted in studies such as those referenced in "Psychoneuroimmunology of Stress and Mental Health" by Dr. George Slavich.[116]

Elevated levels of proinflammatory cytokines, including interleukin-6 (IL-6) and tumor necrosis factor-alpha (TNF-α), have been implicated in the pathogenesis of various chronic diseases, ranging from cardiovascular disorders to autoimmune conditions.

Dr. Sheldon Cohen's investigations into the impact of stress on susceptibility to respiratory infections further underscore the immunosuppressive effects of chronic stress.[117] Individuals experiencing chronic stress exhibit compromised immune responses, leading to increased vulnerability to infections and delayed recovery.

Cardiovascular Consequences of Stress on Heart Health

The cardiovascular system becomes a focal point in the physiological sequelae of chronic stress. Research conducted by Dr. Susan Everson-Rose, as outlined in "Stress and Cardiovascular Disease," establishes a clear association between chronic stress and an elevated risk of cardiovascular diseases.[118]

---

[115] Robert M. Sapolsky, ibid.

[116] George M. Slavich, "Psychoneuroimmunology of Stress and Mental Health," *Psychiatry Clinics of North America*, 2019.

[117] Sheldon Cohen, et al., "Psychological Stress and Susceptibility to the Common Cold," *The New England Journal of Medicine*, 1991.

[118] Susan A. Everson-Rose, et al., "Stress and Cardiovascular Disease," *Journal of the American College of Cardiology*, 2002.

The mechanisms underlying this link involve the interplay of stress-induced hormonal dysregulation, inflammation, and the modulation of autonomic nervous system activity.

The impact of stress on blood pressure regulation further amplifies its significance in cardiovascular health. Dr. Matthew Muldoon's studies underscore the role of chronic stress in elevating blood pressure, predisposing individuals to hypertension—a major risk factor for cardiovascular morbidity and mortality.[119]

Metabolic Implications of Stress on Appetite, and Weight

Chronic stress exerts a profound influence on metabolic pathways, encompassing appetite regulation and weight management. Dr. Elissa Epel's work, as discussed in "The Telomere Effect," explains the impact of stress-induced cortisol release on appetite, emphasizing the link between chronic stress, altered eating behaviors, and the development of obesity.[120]

Insulin resistance, a key feature in the pathogenesis of type 2 diabetes, is closely linked to chronic stress, as well as to the consumption of animal products and other foods high in saturated fats. Dr. Josiane Broussard's research underscores how stress-induced alterations in cortisol levels contribute to insulin resistance, forming a nexus between stress, metabolic dysregulation, and the risk of type 2 diabetes.[121]

In summary, the impact of stress on health transcends psychological distress, prompting detailed physiological processes that span the neuroendocrine, immune, cardiovascular, and metabolic systems.

A comprehensive understanding of these interconnected pathways becomes imperative in formulating effective stress management strategies, underscoring the profound implications of stress on overall health.

---

[119] Matthew F. Muldoon, et al., "Effects of Acute Mental Stress on the Predictability of Risk in Patients With Coronary Artery Disease," *Journal of the American College of Cardiology*, 1999.

[120] Elissa S. Epel and Elizabeth H. Blackburn, "The Telomere Effect: A Revolutionary Approach to Living Younger, Healthier, Longer," Grand Central Publishing, 2017.

[121] Josiane L. Broussard, et al., "Impaired insulin signaling in human adipocytes after experimental sleep restriction: a randomized, crossover study," *Annals of Internal Medicine*, 2012.

PRACTICING MINDFULNESS AND MEDITATION

In the pursuit of effective stress management, the realms of mindfulness and meditation emerge as scientifically validated techniques with far-reaching implications for mental well-being and physiological homeostasis.

Grounded in empirical research, these practices not only mitigate the immediate effects of stress but also induce lasting structural and functional changes in the brain, fostering resilience in the face of adversity.

Mindfulness-Based Stress Reduction (MBSR)

Central to the application of mindfulness in stress management is the Mindfulness-Based Stress Reduction (MBSR) program developed by Dr. Jon Kabat-Zinn. Rooted in the principles outlined in "Full Catastrophe Living," MBSR emphasizes cultivating present-moment awareness through practices such as mindfulness meditation, body scans, and mindful movement.[122]

Scientific investigations into the efficacy of MBSR, as presented in studies like those by Dr. Linda Carlson and Dr. Michael Speca, showcase its effectiveness in reducing stress and improving psychological well-being across diverse populations.[123]

Beyond subjective reports of stress reduction, neuroimaging studies have explored the neural mechanisms underpinning mindfulness practices. For example, Dr. Sara Lazar's work has demonstrated structural changes in brain regions associated with self-awareness, compassion, and cognitive control following mindfulness training.[124]

These neuroplastic changes provide tangible insights into the transformative potential of mindfulness in reshaping the neural architecture implicated in stress processing.

---

[122] Jon Kabat-Zinn, "Full Catastrophe Living: Using the Wisdom of Your Body and Mind to Face Stress, Pain, and Illness," Bantam, 1990.

[123] Linda E. Carlson and Michael R. Speca, "Mindfulness-Based Stress Reduction (MBSR) in Cancer Care: A Systematic Review," *Psycho-Oncology*, 2004.

[124] Sara W. Lazar, et al., "The underlying anatomical correlates of long-term meditation: Larger hippocampal and frontal volumes of gray matter," *NeuroImage*, 2005.

Mindfulness Meditation and the Amygdala

The amygdala, a key hub in the brain's emotional processing network, becomes a focal point in understanding the impact of mindfulness meditation on stress responses.

Dr. J. David Creswell's research, as explored in "Alterations in Brain and Immune Function Produced by Mindfulness Meditation," highlights how mindfulness meditation modulates amygdala reactivity to emotional stimuli, attenuating heightened emotional responses.[125]

Furthermore, studies by Dr. Britta Hölzel explore the functional connectivity changes between the amygdala and regions associated with attention and executive control following mindfulness training.[126]

These connectivity alterations reflect the adaptive recalibration of neural circuits implicated in stress regulation, underscoring the potential of mindfulness meditation in enhancing emotional regulation.

Mindfulness and Cognitive Resilience

Mindfulness practices extend their influence to cortical structures associated with cognitive function and self-awareness. Dr. Amishi Jha's investigations into the impact of mindfulness on attentional control reveal enhanced cognitive resilience in the face of stressors.[127]

Mindfulness training, as explored in studies by Dr. Philippe Goldin and Dr. Elizabeth Hoge, demonstrates improvements in working memory and cognitive flexibility, pivotal components in navigating challenging situations.[128]

---

[125] J. David Creswell, et al., "Alterations in Brain and Immune Function Produced by Mindfulness Meditation," *Psychosomatic Medicine*, 2003.

[126] Britta K. Hölzel, et al., "Mindfulness practice leads to increases in regional brain gray matter density," *Psychiatry Research: Neuroimaging*, 2011.

[127] Amishi P. Jha, et al., "Mindfulness Training Modifies Subsystems of Attention," *Cognitive, Affective, & Behavioral Neuroscience*, 2010.

[128] Philippe, Goldin, et al., "Mindfulness Meditation Training and Self-Referential Processing in Social Anxiety Disorder: Behavioral and Neural Effects", *Journal of Cognitive Psychotherapy*, 2009.

Mindfulness and the Default Mode Network

The Default Mode Network (DMN), implicated in self-referential thinking and mind-wandering, undergoes dynamic shifts during mindfulness meditation.

Dr. Judson Brewer's research elucidates how mindfulness practices deactivate the DMN, reducing self-referential thought patterns associated with rumination and chronic stress.[129]

By fostering a non-judgmental awareness of thoughts and emotions, mindfulness disrupts maladaptive thought patterns, contributing to the alleviation of stress-related psychological symptoms.

Mindful Movement Practices

Mindful movement practices, such as Tai Chi and Yoga, extend the principles of mindfulness to physical activity. Dr. Michael Irwin's investigations into Tai Chi's effects on stress and immune function demonstrate its capacity to modulate stress-related biomarkers and enhance overall well-being.[130]

Similarly, Dr. Sat Bir Khalsa's work on Yoga highlights its efficacy in reducing perceived stress and promoting emotional regulation[131].

In summary, the scientific exploration of mindfulness and meditation unveils their profound impact on stress management—spanning from neuroplastic changes in brain structures to alterations in emotional and cognitive processing.

As individuals incorporate these evidence-based practices into their stress management repertoire, they tap into a reservoir of resilience, reshaping both the mind and body's response to stressors.

---

[129] Judson A. Brewer, et al., "Meditation experience is associated with increased cortical thickness," *NeuroReport*, 2011.

[130] Michael R. Irwin, et al., "Tai Chi and inflammation: A systematic review of randomized controlled trials," *Complementary Therapies in Medicine*, 2019.

[131] Sat Bir S. Khalsa, et al., "Yoga Effects on Brain Health: A Systematic Review of the Current Literature," *Brain Plasticity*, 2019.

DEVELOPING RESILIENCE FOR A LONG AND HEALTHY LIFE

Within the study of human psychology, resilience emerges as a profound force that shapes an individual's response to life's challenges.

Dr. Ann Masten's research, as articulated in "Ordinary Magic: Resilience in Development," delineates resilience as a dynamic interplay of psychological factors, influencing the trajectory of one's well-being with far-reaching implications for long-term health.[132]

Psychological Factors Shaping Resilience

A fundamental aspect of resilience lies in the cultivation of a deep sense of purpose—a guiding force that imbues life with meaning and direction. Dr. Patrick Hill's longitudinal study on purpose in life underscores its impact on health outcomes, revealing that individuals with a clear sense of purpose exhibit better mental health and lower mortality rates.[133]

The social dimension becomes integral to resilience, with positive social connections acting as a pivotal factor. Dr. George Bonanno's extensive work on the social aspects of resilience elucidates the profound impact of supportive relationships.[134] Beyond emotional support, these connections exert a regulatory influence on stress-related physiological responses, offering a buffer against adversities.

Resilient individuals demonstrate a repertoire of adaptive coping strategies, a concept emphasized by Dr. Susan Folkman. Her research underscores the importance of problem-focused coping and emotional regulation in navigating challenges effectively. These strategies empower individuals to confront stressors directly, modulating emotional responses and fostering a resilient mindset.[135]

---

[132] Masten, A. S., "Ordinary Magic: Resilience in Development", 2014.

[133] Hill, P. L., Turiano, N. A., et al., "Purpose in Life as a Predictor of Mortality Across Adulthood." *Psychological Science*, 2016.

[134] Bonanno, G. A., "Resilience in the Face of Potential Trauma.", *Current Directions in Psychological Science*, 2005.

[135] Folkman, S., & Lazarus, R. S., "If It Changes It Must Be a Process: Study of Emotion and Coping During Three Stages of a College Examination." *Journal of Personality and Social Psychology*, 1985.

Post-Traumatic Growth: Transformative Potential in Adversity

The utility of resilience transcends adaptation, encompassing the concept of post-traumatic growth. Dr. Richard Tedeschi and Dr. Lawrence Calhoun's seminal work explores the transformative potential embedded in adversity. Beyond mere adaptation, individuals undergoing challenging experiences can emerge with enhanced psychological well-being, a deeper appreciation for life, and a redefined sense of personal strengths.[136]

Cognitive restructuring becomes a pivotal process within post-traumatic growth, where individuals reassess their priorities, values, and perspectives. Dr. Tedeschi and Dr. Calhoun's exploration reveals that this cognitive shift contributes to a more resilient outlook, influencing responses to future challenges.

A profound appreciation for life, as investigated by Dr. Laura King, becomes a cornerstone of resilience. Cultivating gratitude and savoring positive experiences are identified as factors promoting resilience.[137] This newfound appreciation serves as a psychological resource, contributing to an individual's capacity to navigate life's complexities.

Challenging experiences catalyze not only personal growth but also strengthened relationships. Dr. Sonja Lyubomirsky's research underscores how shared experiences of adversity can deepen interpersonal connections, establishing a resilient support network for future challenges.[138]

As people work on cultivating resilience, mindfulness practices emerge as transformative allies. Dr. Emily Lindsay's research accentuates the link between mindfulness and emotional regulation. These practices foster adaptive responses to stressors, promoting resilience in the face of adversity by modulating emotional reactivity and promoting emotional well-being.[139]

---

[136] Tedeschi, R. G., & Calhoun, L. G., "Posttraumatic Growth: Conceptual Foundations and Empirical Evidence." *Psychological Inquiry,* 2004.

[137] King, L. A., et al., "The Health Benefits of Writing About Life Goals." *Personality and Social Psychology Bulletin,* 2006.

[138] Lyubomirsky, S., et al., "The Benefits of Frequent Positive Affect: Does Happiness Lead to Success?" *Psychological Bulletin*, 2005.

[139] Lindsay, E. K., et al., "Mindfulness Training Alters Emotional Memory Recall Compared to Active Controls: Support for an Emotional Information Processing Model of Mindfulness." *Frontiers in Human Neuroscience,* 2019.

In summary, the cultivation of resilience for a long and healthy life involves a dynamic interplay of psychological factors, including a sense of purpose, positive social connections, adaptive coping strategies, and the transformative potential embedded in adversity.

The integration of these psychological elements, along with the adoption of mindfulness practices, positions individuals on a trajectory toward the enhanced mental and emotional well-being that is conducive to longevity.

CHAPTER 6: THE SOCIAL CONNECTION FACTOR

INTRODUCTION

Within the sphere of human existence and experience, the role of social connections emerges as a pivotal determinant of well-being, influencing not only emotional resilience but also physiological health.

This chapter emphasizes the profound impact on longevity of building and maintaining strong relationships, exploring the scientific underpinnings of how social interactions shape our mental and physical landscape.

The quest for longevity and health intertwines with the quality of our relationships, as evidenced by extensive research in the field of social psychology.

Dr. Julianne Holt-Lunstad's meta-analyses emphasize that individuals with robust social connections exhibit a 50% increased likelihood of longevity compared to those with weaker ties.[140] The reciprocal nature of these relationships plays a key role since the act of providing support is as beneficial as receiving it.

Studies, such as those by Dr. Sheldon Cohen and Dr. Thomas W. Kamarck, illustrate the immunological benefits derived from positive social interactions.[141] The strengthening of the immune system, particularly through enhanced antibody responses, highlights the complex interplay between social connectedness and physiological resilience against pathogens.

The impact of social interactions extends beyond mere survival, however, profoundly influencing mental and emotional well-being. Dr. Ed Diener's research emphasizes the correlation between social support and subjective

---

[140] Julianne Holt-Lunstad, et al., "Social Relationships and Mortality Risk: A Meta-analytic Review," *PLoS Medicine*, 2010.
[141] Sheldon Cohen, et al., "Types of Stressors That Increase Susceptibility to the Common Cold in Healthy Adults," *Health Psychology*, 1998.

well-being, highlighting the role of positive relationships in fostering a sense of life satisfaction.[142]

Moreover, the neurobiological mechanisms engaged during social interactions, as investigated by Dr. Matthew D. Lieberman, shed light on how the brain processes social information and how this processing influences emotional regulation.[143]

Loneliness, conversely, emerges as a risk factor for various health issues. Dr. John T. Cacioppo's work illuminates how chronic loneliness can trigger physiological responses akin to stress, contributing to increased inflammation and compromised immune function.[144]

Understanding the detrimental impact of social isolation underscores the vital role of meaningful connections in preserving both mental and physical health.

The pursuit of a long and healthy life involves not just the presence of social connections but the quality of these relationships. Dr. Robert Waldinger's longitudinal study on adult development at Harvard University underscores the significance of close, emotionally nourishing relationships in promoting happiness and overall life satisfaction.[145] The joy derived from positive social interactions becomes a potent elixir for mental well-being.

Support networks play an important role in navigating life's challenges. Research by Dr. James S. House emphasizes the buffering effect of social support on stress-related health issues, emphasizing how strong social ties contribute to a sense of security and coping resources.[146] The intertwining of emotional support, instrumental assistance, and companionship within social networks becomes a cornerstone in fostering resilience.

In essence, the exploration of the social connection factor unveils the detailed relationship between human bonds and overall health. From the

---

[142] Ed Diener and Martin E. P. Seligman, "Very Happy People," *Psychological Science*, 2002.

[143] Matthew D. Lieberman, "Social: Why Our Brains Are Wired to Connect," *Crown Publishers*, 2013.

[144] John T. Cacioppo, et al., "Loneliness as a Specific Risk Factor for Depressive Symptoms: Cross-sectional and Longitudinal Analyses," *Psychology and Aging*, 2006.

[145] Robert J. Waldinger, et al., "What are the social determinants of positive aging?" *Psychiatric Clinics of North America*, 2013.

[146] James S. House, et al., "Social Relationships and Health," *Science*, 1988.

immunological benefits of positive social interactions to the neurobiological mechanisms underpinning emotional well-being, this chapter aims to unravel the scientific intricacies of our social fabric.

By understanding the profound impact of building strong relationships, recognizing the influence of social interactions on well-being, and finding joy and support in connections, individuals can harness the social connection factor as a potent force in the pursuit of longevity and health.

BUILDING STRONG RELATIONSHIPS

The scientific exploration of human relationships reveals a profound connection between the strength of social bonds and various facets of health, longevity, and well-being.

In the study of social psychology, extensive research underscores the pivotal role that robust relationships play in shaping the human experience.

The Impact of Relationships on Longevity

Dr. Julianne Holt-Lunstad's influential meta-analyses have demonstrated a compelling link between the quality of social connections and longevity. Individuals with strong social ties exhibit a remarkable 50% increased likelihood of prolonged survival when compared to those with weaker connections.[147]

This association is not solely attributable to emotional support but extends to tangible health benefits, indicating a systemic influence of social bonds on physiological resilience.

The reciprocal nature of social relationships proves pivotal in this context. Providing support to others, an integral component of strong relationships, is revealed as a contributing factor to enhanced well-being.

The act of giving support has been associated with reduced mortality rates, highlighting the bidirectional impact of interpersonal connections.[148]

---

[147] Julianne Holt-Lunstad, et al., "Social Relationships and Mortality Risk: A Meta-analytic Review," *PLoS Medicine*, 2010.
[148] Julianne Holt-Lunstad, et al., ibid.

Immunological Benefits of Positive Social Interactions

Positive social interactions trigger immunological responses that contribute to the overall resilience of the human body. Studies led by Dr. Sheldon Cohen and Dr. Thomas W. Kamarck have illuminated how such interactions, marked by emotional support and camaraderie, enhance immune function.[149]

Strengthened antibody responses and heightened immunological defenses serve as tangible markers of the complex interplay between social connectedness and physiological well-being.

Processing Social Information via Neurobiological Mechanisms

The influence of strong relationships extends beyond the physiological realm to complex neurobiological mechanisms. Dr. Matthew D. Lieberman's work explores how the brain processes social information and regulates emotional responses during social interactions.[150]

Understanding the neural underpinnings of social connections provides insights into the role of these bonds in emotional regulation, stress mitigation, and overall mental health.

Coping Resources and Security

Dr. James S. House's research underscores the multifaceted nature of social support by emphasizing its buffering effect on stress-related health issues.[151] Strong social ties serve as reservoirs of coping resources, offering individuals a sense of security and emotional well-being when facing life's challenges.

The intertwining of emotional support, instrumental assistance, and companionship within social networks becomes essential in fostering resilience and adapting to stressors.

---

[149] Sheldon Cohen, et al., "Types of Stressors That Increase Susceptibility to the Common Cold in Healthy Adults," *Health Psychology*, 1998.
[150] Matthew D. Lieberman, "Social: Why Our Brains Are Wired to Connect," *Crown Publishers*, 2013.
[151] James S. House, et al., "Social Relationships and Health," *Science*, 1988.

In summary, building strong relationships is not merely a subjective aspect of human experience; it is deeply interwoven with objective indicators of health and well-being.

From the demonstrable impact on longevity to the immunological benefits of positive social interactions and the neurobiological mechanisms regulating emotional responses, the scientific exploration of social connections underscores their vital role in supporting human health.

SOCIAL INTERACTIONS INFLUENCE WELL-BEING

Exploring the realm of social psychology unveils the profound impact of social interactions on the multifaceted dimensions of human well-being.

The scientific study of these dynamics consistently underscores the detailed interplay between social bonds and mental, emotional, and physical health.

Subjective Well-Being and Social Support

Dr. Ed Diener's research illuminates a robust correlation between social support and subjective well-being.[152] Positive relationships, marked by emotional and instrumental support, contribute significantly to an individual's sense of life satisfaction. The quality of these connections becomes a determining factor in fostering a positive psychological outlook and emotional resilience.

Neurobiological investigations, as undertaken by Dr. Matthew D. Lieberman, have explored the brain's processing of social information to reveal how positive social interactions regulate emotional responses.[153] This neurobiological perspective sheds light on the complex mechanisms through which social interactions contribute to emotional well-being.

The Role of Social Information Processing in Emotional Regulation

Understanding the brain's processing of social information unveils its key role in emotional regulation. Dr. Lieberman's work emphasizes that social

---

[152] Ed Diener and Martin E. P. Seligman, "Very Happy People," *Psychological Science*, 2002.

[153] Matthew D. Lieberman, "Social: Why Our Brains Are Wired to Connect," *Crown Publishers*, 2013.

interactions serve as a regulatory mechanism, influencing emotional responses and mitigating the impact of stressors.[154]

The neurobiological intricacies of social information processing highlight the profound influence of these interactions on an individual's overall emotional experience.

Loneliness and its Adverse Impact on Health

Conversely, chronic loneliness emerges as a risk factor for various health issues. Dr. John T. Cacioppo's extensive research delineates how loneliness triggers physiological responses akin to stress, contributing to increased inflammation and compromised immune function.[155]

This underscores the detailed connection between social isolation and physiological well-being, with loneliness acting as a significant determinant.

The Neurobiology of Social Interaction and Emotional Regulation

Neurobiological investigations, such as those exploring the Default Mode Network (DMN), provide insights into the brain's engagement during social interactions[2]. The DMN, implicated in self-referential thinking, undergoes dynamic shifts during social engagement.

Dr. Judson A. Brewer's work accentuates how social interactions, particularly those characterized by mindfulness and presence, disrupt maladaptive thought patterns, contributing to the alleviation of stress-related psychological symptoms.[156]

Social Support's Overall Impact on Mental and Emotional Health

In essence, the influence of social interactions on well-being spans across subjective, emotional, and even neurobiological dimensions. Positive social support fosters subjective well-being, offering a buffer against the adversities of life.

---

[154] Matthew D. Lieberman, "Social: Why Our Brains Are Wired to Connect," *Crown Publishers*, 2013.

[155] John T. Cacioppo, et al., "Loneliness as a Specific Risk Factor for Depressive Symptoms: Cross-sectional and Longitudinal Analyses," *Psychology and Aging*, 2006.

[156] Judson A. Brewer, et al., "Meditation experience is associated with increased cortical thickness," *NeuroReport*, 2011.

Simultaneously, the neurobiological underpinnings of social information processing shed light on the complex mechanisms through which social interactions regulate emotional responses, contributing to overall mental health.

Understanding the impact of social interactions on well-being becomes a pivotal aspect of the broader exploration into the social connection factor. By unraveling the scientific intricacies of these dynamics, individuals can recognize the profound influence that positive social bonds exert on their mental and emotional landscapes.

FINDING SUPPORT AND HAPPINESS IN CONNECTIONS

The complex nature of human connections extends beyond mere associations, encapsulating profound implications for well-being, resilience, and overall life satisfaction.

This section discusses the importance of finding support and joy within social connections to well-being and longevity, revealing the nuanced dynamics that contribute to a fulfilling and health-promoting social life.

The Role of Emotional Nourishment

Building on the longitudinal study of adult development at Harvard University by Dr. Robert J. Waldinger and his colleagues, it becomes evident that close, emotionally nourishing relationships significantly contribute to happiness and overall life satisfaction.[157]

Beyond the surface level of social interaction, these connections provide a profound sense of emotional support and companionship, essential components in navigating life's challenges.

Happiness Derived from Positive Social Interactions

Positive social interactions become a potent source of happiness, influencing both emotional and physiological aspects of well-being. Dr. Ed Diener's research highlights the correlation between positive relationships

---

[157] Robert J. Waldinger, et al., "What are the social determinants of positive aging?" *Psychiatric Clinics of North America*, 2013.

and subjective well-being, emphasizing the joy derived from meaningful connections.[158]

The reciprocal nature of the experience of happiness within social bonds underscores the importance of fostering positive interactions for sustained mental and emotional health.

The Multifaceted Nature of Social Support

The concept of social support spans a spectrum of forms, encompassing emotional, instrumental, and informational dimensions. Dr. James S. House's seminal work emphasizes the multifaceted nature of social support and its key role in buffering the impact of stress-related health issues.[159]

Emotional support provides solace during challenging times, instrumental support offers tangible assistance, and informational support equips individuals with valuable knowledge—cumulatively contributing to a resilient foundation.

Happiness and Social Hormones

Scientific investigations into the neurobiological mechanisms of joy within social connections reveal the involvement of social hormones. Oxytocin, often referred to as the "bonding hormone," is released during positive social interactions and has been linked to increased feelings of trust and bonding[2].

The interplay between feelings of happiness, social connections, and the release of these hormones underscores the detailed physiological responses that accompany positive social experiences.

The Reciprocal Nature of Support

An essential aspect of deriving support and happiness from social connections lies in the reciprocal nature of these relationships. Providing support to others, as explored in Dr. Julianne Holt-Lunstad's research, is not only beneficial for the recipient but also contributes to the provider's well-being.[160]

---

[158] Ed Diener and Martin E. P. Seligman, "Very Happy People," *Psychological Science*, 2002.

[159] James S. House, et al., "Social Relationships and Health," *Science*, 1988.

This reciprocal dynamic reinforces the notion that happiness and support within social connections are symbiotic, creating a positive feedback loop.

Conclusion

In summary, finding support and joy within social connections transcends the superficial realm of interactions. It involves experiencing the emotional nourishment derived from close relationships, the fundamental pleasure embedded in experiencing positive social interactions, and the multifaceted nature of social support.

This exploration intertwines with neurobiological mechanisms and hormonal responses, offering a comprehensive understanding of the profound impact that meaningful social bonds can exert on individual well-being.

---

[160] Julianne Holt-Lunstad, et al., "Social Relationships and Mortality Risk: A Meta-analytic Review," *PLoS Medicine*, 2010.

74

CHAPTER 7: BREAKING HARMFUL SUBSTANCE USE HABITS FOR A HEALTHIER FUTURE

INTRODUCTION

In the pursuit of longevity and a robust state of health, the impact of harmful substance use habits cannot be overstated. This chapter serves as a scientific guide, delving into the intricacies of eliminating alcohol intake, quitting smoking, avoiding harmful drug use, and overcoming addictions.

Grounded in evidence-based research and clinical insights, the exploration aims to empower individuals to break free from detrimental substance use habits, fostering a path towards a healthier and more resilient future.

This chapter's section on eliminating alcohol intake navigates the complexities of alcohol consumption's impact on health. Drawing from studies such as those by Dr. Jürgen Rehm and his colleagues, we explore the nuanced relationship between alcohol consumption and various health outcomes.[161]

From liver diseases to brain damage to cardiovascular complications, understanding the scientific underpinnings of the harm alcohol consumption causes provides a foundation for individuals seeking to eliminate alcohol intake and enhance their overall well-being.

Furthermore, quitting smoking tobacco stands as a clear transformative step towards better health since the poisonous herb kills a third of its regular users. This section examines the physiological and psychological aspects of nicotine addiction, referencing authoritative sources like the work of Dr. Michael Fiore and Dr. Richard Hurt.[162]

---

[161] Jürgen Rehm, et al., "Global burden of disease and injury and economic cost attributable to alcohol use and alcohol-use disorders," *The Lancet*, 2009.
[162] Michael C. Fiore and Richard D. Hurt, "Treating Tobacco Use and Dependence: An Introduction," *Respiratory Care*, 2000.

By unraveling the mechanisms of nicotine addiction and elucidating effective cessation strategies, individuals can embark on a healthier path toward a smoke-free future.

The section advocating for avoiding harmful drug use extends beyond common substances to encompass a spectrum of pharmacological agents. Authorities like the National Institute on Drug Abuse (NIDA) and the World Health Organization (WHO) provide insights into the consequences of drug misuse.[163] This section equips readers with a comprehensive understanding of the risks associated with various drugs, enabling informed decisions and preventive measures.

The final section of this chapter will discuss methods for overcoming addictions. Drawing on research from addiction medicine experts like Dr. Nora D. Volkow, we will explore the neurological aspects of addiction and evidence-based interventions.[164] Understanding the neural pathways involved in addiction and the potential for neuroplasticity opens avenues for effective interventions and long-term recovery.

In essence, this chapter synthesizes scientific knowledge to offer a roadmap for breaking harmful substance use habits. From the physiological effects of alcohol on the liver to the complexities of nicotine addiction, the exploration encompasses a breadth of substances and their impact on health. By empowering individuals with evidence-based insights, this chapter aims to catalyze positive change, fostering a healthier and more resilient future.

ELIMINATING ALCOHOL INTAKE

The decision to eliminate alcohol intake is a critical step towards enhancing both physical and mental well-being with substantial benefits for longevity in most cases.

---

[163] World Health Organization (WHO), "Management of Substance Abuse: Information Sheet," 2021.

[164] Nora D. Volkow, et al., "Dopamine in Drug Abuse and Addiction: Results from Imaging Studies and Treatment Implications," *Molecular Psychiatry*, 2009.

The ramifications of alcohol consumption extend far beyond social contexts, with its adverse effects spanning physiological, psychological, and interpersonal dimensions.

In this section, we navigate the scientific intricacies of the impact of alcohol on health, exploring the imperative of eliminating its intake for a healthier future.

Alcohol-Related Mortality

Alcohol-related issues contribute significantly to global mortality, with millions of lives affected annually. According to comprehensive studies, including those conducted by the World Health Organization (WHO), alcohol use is linked to approximately 3 million deaths worldwide each year.[165]

This staggering figure underscores the urgent need for awareness and action to address the public health challenges associated with alcohol consumption.

Organ Damage Caused to the Liver, Pancreas, and Brain

The liver stands as a primary target of alcohol-induced damage. Chronic alcohol use can lead to liver inflammation, fatty liver disease, and, in severe cases, cirrhosis.

Research, such as that by Dr. Howard J. Worman, highlights the complex mechanisms through which alcohol metabolism contributes to liver pathology.[166] Understanding these processes becomes pivotal for individuals aiming to eliminate alcohol intake and preserve liver function.

Moreover, the pancreas bears the brunt of alcohol-related harm, as exemplified by studies like those conducted by Dr. Julia Mayerle and her colleagues.[167] Chronic alcohol consumption heightens the risk of pancreatitis, disrupting digestive processes and inducing significant discomfort.

The neurological toll on the human brain of alcohol use is equally profound, with alcohol's impact on the brain elucidated by research such as

---

[165] World Health Organization (WHO), "Alcohol," 2021

[166] Howard J. Worman, "Alcohol and the Liver," *Clinics in Liver Disease*, 2005.

[167] Julia Mayerle, et al., "Chronic alcohol consumption induces pancreatic oxidative damage in rats," *Pancreatology*, 2007.

that conducted by Dr. Reisa A. Sperling.[168] Beyond general cognitive impairments experienced while under the influence of alcohol, alcohol use also inflicts specific damage on brain executive functions.

These key functions, responsible for higher-level cognitive processes like decision-making, planning, and impulse control, become compromised with chronic alcohol intake.[169]

Understanding the direct link between alcohol use and executive function damage emphasizes the critical role of eliminating alcohol for the preservation of cognitive health and the key ability to organize your life effectively.

Alcohol's Impact on Relationships and Safety

Beyond the serious physiological consequences, alcohol use can exert a substantial toll on interpersonal relationships. The influence of alcohol on mood, behavior, and decision-making is well-documented, contributing to conflicts within relationships. The work of Dr. Kenneth E. Leonard and Dr. Sarah E. Ullman sheds light on the complex dynamics between alcohol use and relationship distress.[170]

Safety concerns further underscore the imperative of eliminating alcohol intake. Alcohol impairs cognitive functions and motor skills, significantly increasing the risk of accidents and injuries. Studies, such as those by Dr. Timothy Naimi and colleagues, highlight the link between alcohol consumption and various forms of unintentional injuries.[171] The decision to abstain from alcohol is thus a fundamental step towards ensuring personal safety and the safety of others.

In conclusion, eliminating alcohol intake emerges as a cornerstone in the pursuit of a healthier future. The global magnitude of alcohol-related mortality, coupled with the detailed physiological damage to organs and

---

[168] Reisa A. Sperling, "Alcohol and the Central Nervous System," *Journal of Neuropsychiatry and Clinical Neurosciences*, 2012.

[169] Oscar-Berman, M., & Marinković, K. (2003). Alcoholism and the brain: an overview. *Alcohol research & health, 27*(2), 125–133.

[170] Kenneth E. Leonard and Sarah E. Ullman, "Alcohol and intimate partner violence: when can we say that heavy drinking is a contributing cause of violence?" *Addiction*, 2019.

[171] Timothy Naimi, et al., "Fatal injury attributed to alcohol use in the United States," *Addiction*, 2017.

specific harm to brain executive functions, underscores the imperative of informed and decisive action.

Beyond individual well-being, the impact on relationships and safety highlights the broader societal implications of alcohol consumption. By synthesizing scientific insights, this section aims to empower individuals with the knowledge needed to make informed choices for a healthier and more resilient life.

QUITTING SMOKING

If you smoke tobacco, then the decision to quit smoking is a profound commitment to safeguarding both your individual and public health.

Tobacco smoking remains a leading cause of preventable diseases, exerting a substantial toll on the well-being of millions. Not only does tobacco ultimately kill a third of its users, but it kills roughly half of those who fail to quit the deadly habit that can also adversely impact the health of non-smokers exposed to second-hand tobacco smoke.

This section explains how tobacco smoking harms human health to clarify just how urgent the imperative of quitting smoking is if you desire a healthier future.

Tobacco-Related Mortality is a Global Epidemic

The profound impact of tobacco smoking on global mortality is a stark reality. According to extensive research, including reports from the World Health Organization (WHO), tobacco use is responsible for over 8 million deaths annually.[172]

Alarmingly, the Centers for Disease Control and Prevention (CDC) reports that a third of its users succumb to tobacco-related diseases, emphasizing the lethal nature of this pervasive, addictive, and remarkably unhealthy habit.[173]

---

[172] World Health Organization (WHO), "Tobacco," 2021.
[173] Centers for Disease Control and Prevention (CDC), "Fast Facts," 2021.

This staggering death toll underscores the urgency of quitting smoking as a fundamental step towards extending human longevity and mitigating the global burden of preventable diseases.

Tobacco Use Shortens Your Expected Lifespan

The detrimental impact of tobacco on human lifespan is unequivocal, with extensive research highlighting the stark reality of premature mortality associated with smoking. Studies, including comprehensive analyses conducted by organizations such as the American Cancer Society, consistently reveal that tobacco use significantly shortens a person's lifespan.

On average, smokers face a substantially higher risk of premature death compared to non-smokers, with estimates suggesting that smoking can reduce lifespan by an alarming average of 10 years.[174]

The toxic cocktail of chemicals in tobacco smoke not only heightens the vulnerability to a myriad of life-threatening illnesses, including cancer, cardiovascular diseases, and respiratory conditions but also accelerates the aging process at the cellular level.

Components of tobacco also compete with vitamin C, making it unusually harmful to your immune system that protects you from infections and other illnesses.

Understanding the profound adverse impact of tobacco use on longevity underscores the urgency of quitting smoking for individuals seeking to reclaim a healthier and more extended life.

Health and Physiological Consequences of Tobacco Use

Smoking tobacco inflicts severe damage on the respiratory system. Chronic exposure to tobacco smoke is a primary driver of conditions such as chronic bronchitis and emphysema. Quitting smoking thus becomes pivotal in halting the progression of these debilitating respiratory conditions.

---

[174] American Cancer Society, "How Tobacco Smoke Causes Disease: The Biology and Behavioral Basis for Smoking-Attributable Disease," 2010.

The interaction between tobacco smoke and the respiratory epithelium, as explored in studies like those conducted by Dr. Peter J. Barnes, reveals the underlying mechanisms of chronic obstructive pulmonary disease (COPD).[175]

Beyond the lungs, tobacco smoking poses formidable risks to cardiovascular health. Extensive research, including that of Dr. Stanton A. Glantz, emphasizes the correlation between smoking and coronary heart disease, stroke, and peripheral vascular disease.[176]

The detrimental impact on blood vessels, driven by the complex interplay of the toxins contained in tobacco smoke, underscores the urgency of quitting smoking to mitigate cardiovascular risks.

The Neurobiological Grip of Nicotine Addiction

Central to the challenge of quitting smoking is the neurobiological grip of nicotine addiction. Nicotine, the addictive component of tobacco, exerts its influence on the brain's reward pathways, contributing to cravings and withdrawal symptoms.

Furthermore, Dr. Nora D. Volkow's research into the complex neurobiology of nicotine addiction emphasizes the need for comprehensive interventions to break free from its grasp.[177]

Understanding the neurobiological underpinnings becomes paramount for individuals aiming to quit smoking successfully.

Secondhand Smoke is a Public Health Concern

Quitting smoking not only benefits the individual but also plays a key role in mitigating the impact of secondhand smoke on other people in your life and public health in general.

The work of Dr. Jonathan M. Samet and others highlights the association between secondhand smoke exposure and adverse health outcomes, particularly in nonsmokers.[178]

---

[175] Peter J. Barnes, "Chronic Obstructive Pulmonary Disease: Effects beyond the Lungs," *PLOS Medicine*, 2010.

[176] Stanton A. Glantz, "Meta-analysis of the effects of secondhand smoke exposure on stroke and coronary heart disease," *Circulation*, 2006.

[177] Nora D. Volkow, et al., "Dopamine in Drug Abuse and Addiction: Results from Imaging Studies and Treatment Implications," *Molecular Psychiatry*, 2009.

By quitting smoking, individuals contribute not only to their well-being but also to creating smoke-free environments that protect the health of those around them.

In conclusion, quitting smoking stands as a key way to improve both individual and public health. The global epidemic of tobacco-related mortality, coupled with the harsh physiological consequences and the neurobiological challenges of nicotine addiction, underscores the urgency of embracing a smoke-free future.

By synthesizing scientific insights, this section aims to empower individuals with the knowledge needed to overcome the grip of tobacco smoking and transition towards a healthier and more resilient life.

Strategies for Quitting Tobacco

The path to quit smoking demands a multifaceted approach, harnessing various strategies to address both the physical and psychological dimensions of nicotine addiction.

While the grip of tobacco can be formidable since nicotine has the highest addictiveness potential of virtually any known substance, individuals can employ diverse methods to enhance their chances of successfully breaking free from this harmful habit. Some of those methods include:

Hypnotherapy:

Hypnotherapy, under the guidance of trained professionals, taps into the power of suggestion to reshape subconscious patterns associated with smoking. Studies, such as those conducted by Dr. Timothy P. Carmody, suggest that hypnotherapy can be a valuable adjunct to traditional smoking cessation interventions, enhancing quit rates.[179]

By addressing the psychological aspects of addiction, hypnotherapy provides individuals with a tool to navigate cravings and reinforce their commitment to a smoke-free life.

Behavioral Therapies:

---

[178] Jonathan M. Samet, "The Health Benefits of Smoking Cessation," *Medicine & Health/Rhode Island*, 2009.

[179] Timothy P. Carmody, et al., "Hypnosis for Smoking Cessation: A Randomized Trial," *Nicotine & Tobacco Research*, 2008.

Behavioral therapies, including cognitive-behavioral therapy (CBT), offer effective strategies for modifying the thoughts and behaviors intertwined with smoking.

Dr. Saul Shiffman's research highlights the efficacy of behavioral interventions in smoking cessation, emphasizing the importance of addressing the habitual aspects of tobacco use.[180]

By identifying triggers and developing coping mechanisms, individuals can gradually dismantle the associations that sustain smoking behavior.

Pharmacotherapy:

Pharmacotherapeutic approaches, such as nicotine replacement therapy (NRT) and prescription medications like varenicline, provide physiological support in managing withdrawal symptoms.

Dr. Michael C. Fiore's extensive work on smoking cessation pharmacotherapy underscores the value of these interventions in mitigating the challenges of nicotine dependence.[181]

These options offer a structured pathway for individuals looking to alleviate the physiological aspects of addiction.

Supportive Networks:

Building a robust support network is pivotal in the process of quitting smoking. Engaging with support groups, whether in-person or online, fosters a sense of community and shared commitment.

Research, including studies by Dr. Amanda L. Graham, emphasizes the positive impact of social support on smoking cessation outcomes.[182]

Sharing experiences, setbacks, and successes with peers provides valuable insights and encouragement throughout the quitting process.

---

[180] Saul Shiffman, et al., "Efficacy of nicotine lozenge for smoking cessation," Addiction, 2002.

[181] Michael C. Fiore, et al., "Treating Tobacco Use and Dependence: An Introduction," Respiratory Care, 2000.

[182] Amanda L. Graham, et al., "Effectiveness of an Internet-Based Worksite Smoking Cessation Intervention at 12 Months," Journal of Occupational and Environmental Medicine, 2007.

Start Quitting Tobacco Now

In summary, tobacco use is deadly and clearly counterproductive to anyone wishing to extend their lifespan. While the path to quitting smoking is diverse, it reflects the unique needs and preferences of individuals aiming to improve their health and longevity by eliminating tobacco use from their lives.

By integrating strategies like hypnotherapy, behavioral therapies, pharmacotherapy, and supportive networks, individuals can bolster their arsenal against tobacco dependence.

Using a combination of these approaches may help address the physical and psychological factors in tobacco addiction, offering a comprehensive framework for a successful and enduring transition to a healthier smoke-free life and longer life.

AVOID HARMFUL DRUG USE

The imperative to cultivate a healthier future extends to avoiding the pitfalls of harmful drug use, recognizing the severe physical, mental, and societal repercussions associated with the excessive use of certain substances.

While acknowledging the relative harmlessness of recreational drugs like cannabis and the psychedelics, it is paramount to address the detrimental impact of highly addictive and potentially dangerous drugs such as cocaine, heroin, and methamphetamine that can all cause deadly overdoses and health disruptions.

Scientific evidence underscores the imperative of steering clear of these substances for the preservation of individual well-being and public health.

Cocaine: A Risky Stimulant

Cocaine, a powerful stimulant derived from the coca plant, poses profound risks to health. Extensive research, including studies by Dr. Richard Rawson, highlights the acute cardiovascular consequences of cocaine use, ranging from elevated heart rate and blood pressure to increased risk of heart attacks and strokes.[183]

The addictive nature of cocaine further exacerbates these health risks, leading to a cycle of dependence that can have lasting, detrimental effects on both physical and mental health.

Heroin: An Opioid Epidemic

Heroin, an opioid derived from morphine, stands at the epicenter of a devastating global epidemic. Dr. Nora D. Volkow's research illuminates the neurobiological impact of heroin, underscoring its potential to alter brain circuits associated with judgment and decision-making.[184]

The risk of overdose and the transmission of infectious diseases through needle sharing compound the severe health hazards associated with heroin use, demanding a comprehensive approach to address the multifaceted challenges posed by this highly addictive substance.

Methamphetamine: A Stimulating Health Menace

Methamphetamine, a potent central nervous system stimulant, inflicts profound harm on physical and mental well-being. Research, such as that conducted by Dr. Richard A. Rawson, outlines the neurotoxic effects of methamphetamine on the brain, leading to cognitive deficits and emotional disturbances.[185]

The heightened risk of addiction and the associated impact on individuals and communities necessitate concerted efforts to discourage the use of methamphetamine for the sake of public health and longevity.

Pharmaceutical Drug Use Can Also Harm Your Health

Beyond recreational substances, the cautious use of pharmaceutical drugs is equally imperative. While many pharmaceuticals bring therapeutic benefits, their misuse or abuse can lead to severe health consequences.

---

[183] Richard Rawson, et al., "Cardiovascular effects of the methylecgonidine crack cocaine," *Journal of Cardiovascular Pharmacology and Therapeutics*, 2012.
[184] Nora D. Volkow, et al., "Imaging the Addicted Brain: Insights from Neuroimaging of Opioid Use Disorders," *The American Journal of Psychiatry*, 2017.
[185] Richard A. Rawson, "Neurotoxicity of Methamphetamine: A Review of Recent Findings," *Current Pharmaceutical Design*, 2012.

Some pharmaceutical drugs can also have severe side effects, including death, so read warning labels, look for safer alternatives, and watch out for adverse reactions if you do decide to take pharmaceutical drugs on the advice of a medical professional.

Dr. Aaron M. Gilson's work emphasizes the risks associated with the nonmedical use of prescription drugs, with opioid analgesics being a notable example.[186]

Striking a balance between legitimate medical use and preventing the potential for addiction and adverse health outcomes requires a nuanced approach to pharmaceutical drug usage.

Using Harmful Drugs May Harm Your Health and Shorten Your Life

In conclusion, the pursuit of a healthier future demands a steadfast commitment to avoiding harmful drug use, recognizing the distinct risks posed by substances like cocaine, heroin, and methamphetamine.

By leveraging scientific insights, individuals can make informed choices that prioritize both individual well-being and the broader fabric of societal health.

OVERCOMING ADDICTIONS FOR A HEALTHIER FUTURE

The path toward a healthier future necessitates a nuanced understanding of addiction and a comprehensive approach to break the chains that bind individuals to harmful substances.

The following subsections explore preventive measures to avoid addiction and effective methods for quitting substance use.

Preventive Measures: Avoiding Addiction

A foundational aspect of preventing addiction lies in arming individuals with comprehensive knowledge about substances and their appropriate and moderate use.

---

[186] Aaron M. Gilson, et al., "Nonmedical use of prescription opioids among teenagers in the United States: trends and correlates," Journal of Adolescent Health, 2012.

Dr. Nora D. Volkow's pioneering research elucidates the neurobiological underpinnings of addiction, emphasizing the critical role of education in dissuading individuals from initiating substance use.[187]

By fostering awareness of the potential consequences, individuals can make better and more informed decisions that prioritize their long-term health over immediate gratification.

Cognitive-Behavioral Strategies:

The application of cognitive-behavioral strategies, explored extensively in studies such as those by Dr. Alan Marlatt, provides individuals with effective tools to prevent and interrupt addictive behaviors.[188]

These strategies target thought patterns and behaviors associated with substance use, empowering individuals to identify triggers and develop coping mechanisms. By addressing underlying factors, cognitive-behavioral strategies serve as a proactive measure against the onset of addiction.

Effective Methods for Quitting Substance Use

In cases where addiction has taken root, pharmacotherapy emerges as a helpful component of the recovery process. Medications like buprenorphine and methadone, highlighted in the work of Dr. George E. Woody, play a pivotal role in managing opioid addiction by mitigating cravings and withdrawal symptoms.[189] Integrating pharmacotherapy into comprehensive treatment plans enhances the potential for successful recovery.

Behavioral interventions, including contingency management and motivational enhancement therapy, have also demonstrated efficacy in promoting abstinence from substance use.[190] Dr. Nancy M. Petry's research underscores the positive impact of these interventions in reinforcing pro-recovery behaviors and enhancing treatment outcomes. By addressing

---

[187] Nora D. Volkow, et al., "The Addicted Human Brain: Insights from Imaging Studies," *Journal of Clinical Investigation*, 2003.

[188] Alan Marlatt, "Harm Reduction: Come as You Are," *Addiction*, 1996.

[189] George E. Woody, et al., "Extended vs short-term buprenorphine-naloxone for treatment of opioid-addicted youth: a randomized trial," *JAMA*, 2008.

[190] Nancy M. Petry, "A comprehensive guide to the application of contingency management procedures in clinical settings," *Drug and Alcohol Dependence*, 2000.

psychological aspects and reinforcing positive behaviors, behavioral interventions contribute significantly to the recovery process.

Furthermore, building and leveraging supportive networks is fundamental to overcoming addiction. Dr. Keith Humphreys' research emphasizes the role of social support in sustaining recovery and reducing the risk of relapse.[191] Engaging with support groups, therapy, and community resources provides individuals with the encouragement and understanding needed to navigate the challenges of addiction recovery. The communal strength derived from these networks proves instrumental in fostering resilience and commitment to a substance-free life.

Finally, understanding the concept of neuroplasticity is integral to addiction recovery. Dr. Nora D. Volkow's research sheds light on the brain's capacity to rewire itself, offering hope for recovery through sustained abstinence from addictive substances.[192] Engaging in activities that promote neuroplasticity, such as cognitive exercises and mindfulness practices, becomes a cornerstone of the healing process, allowing the brain to adapt and heal.

In conclusion, overcoming addiction is generally a multifaceted endeavor that demands a strategic blend of preventive measures and effective intervention methods.

By combining informed decision-making, pharmacotherapy, behavioral interventions, supportive networks, and an understanding of neuroplasticity, individuals can navigate the challenging path toward lasting recovery and a healthier future.

---

[191] Keith Humphreys, et al., "Friendship and supportive relationships in recovery: Composing a good life," *Addiction Research & Theory*, 2018.

[192] Nora D. Volkow, et al., "Neurobiologic Advances from the Brain Disease Model of Addiction," *New England Journal of Medicine*, 2016.

CHAPTER 8: GET REGULAR HEALTH CHECK-UPS

INTRODUCTION

Embarking on a path towards optimal health as you age requires a proactive commitment to regular health check-ups. This pivotal chapter explores the multifaceted benefits of monitoring one's health, encompassing key disease prevention methods, early detection strategies, and the importance of collaborating with healthcare professionals.

Rooted in scientific evidence and expert insights, this chapter underscores the paramount importance of regular health assessments in safeguarding well-being.

Scientific research, such as studies conducted by Dr. Russell Harris and Dr. Michael Pignone, illuminates the vital role of health monitoring in preventing and managing chronic diseases.[193]

Regular health check-ups serve as a cornerstone for assessing risk factors, monitoring vital signs, and identifying early indicators of potential health issues.

The proactive approach of regular monitoring empowers individuals to make informed decisions about lifestyle and preventive measures, ultimately contributing to the maintenance of long-term health.

Furthermore, prevention lies at the heart of sustained well-being. Dr. David L. Katz's extensive work on preventive medicine highlights the significance of adopting a comprehensive approach to disease prevention.[194]

The section on this topic looks into some evidence-based preventive methods, including lifestyle modifications, vaccinations, and tailored

---

[193] Russell Harris, et al., "Screening for colorectal cancer: systematic review," *JAMA*, 2008.

[194] David L. Katz, et al., "Preventive Medicine, Integrative Medicine & the Health of the Public," *American Journal of Preventive Medicine*, 2015.

interventions, providing readers with actionable insights to mitigate the risk of various health conditions.

In addition, early detection of disease forms a critical component of an effective healthcare strategy. Research by organizations such as the American Cancer Society emphasizes the impact of timely screenings and diagnostic tests in detecting diseases at their nascent stages.[195]

The section on this topic will explore the science behind early disease detection, elucidating how routine health check-ups can facilitate the identification of anomalies before they progress, offering individuals a greater chance of successful intervention and treatment.

Finally, the collaborative relationship between individuals and healthcare professionals is pivotal in maintaining and enhancing health. Dr. Eric Topol's work emphasizes the transformative potential of patient-centered care and collaborative decision-making.[196]

The section on this topic will explore the dynamics of effective collaboration, providing guidance on communication, shared decision-making, and leveraging the expertise of healthcare professionals to tailor personalized health plans.

In essence, this chapter offers a comprehensive guide to fostering a proactive approach to health that will keep you looking younger and feeling healthier well into your golden years.

By exploring the importance of health monitoring, disease prevention methods, early detection strategies, and collaborative healthcare partnerships, this chapter equips readers with the knowledge and tools needed to prioritize their well-being.

THE IMPORTANCE OF MONITORING YOUR HEALTH

Regular health check-ups stand as a fundamental pillar in the pursuit of optimal well-being, rooted in the scientific understanding that proactive monitoring can significantly impact disease prevention and early

---

[195] American Cancer Society, "Cancer Facts & Figures 2021," 2021.
[196] Eric Topol, "The Patient Will See You Now: The Future of Medicine is in Your Hands," 2015.

intervention. This section explores the multifaceted significance of health monitoring, drawing upon insights from studies and experts in the field.

Risk Assessment and Early Intervention

Health monitoring enables a comprehensive assessment of individual health risks. Studies, such as those by Dr. Michael Pignone and Dr. Russell Harris, emphasize the importance of risk assessment in guiding preventive measures.[197]

Through regular check-ups, individuals gain valuable insights into factors such as blood pressure, cholesterol levels, and blood glucose, allowing for the early identification of potential risk factors associated with cardiovascular diseases and diabetes.

This, in turn, empowers individuals to adopt timely interventions, whether through lifestyle modifications or medical interventions.

Detecting Silent Conditions

Certain health conditions may manifest silently, without overt symptoms. Routine health assessments serve as a vital tool in unearthing these hidden conditions.

Dr. Robert W. Haley's research underscores the importance of regular health screenings in detecting silent killers, such as hypertension, which may otherwise go unnoticed.[198]

By uncovering these conditions early on, individuals can initiate appropriate management strategies, mitigating the risk of complications and enhancing overall health outcomes.

Monitoring Chronic Conditions

For individuals managing chronic conditions, regular health check-ups play a pivotal role in disease management.

---

[197] Michael Pignone, et al., "Screening and Interventions for Unhealthy Alcohol Use in Primary Care Settings: A Clinical Practice Guideline," *JAMA*, 2020.
[198] Robert W. Haley, "Effectiveness of Routine Vaccination in Reversing Declines in Invasive Streptococcus pneumoniae Infections," *The American Journal of Medicine*, 2010.

Dr. Eric Topol's insights into patient-centered care highlight the collaborative relationship between individuals and healthcare professionals in monitoring chronic conditions.[199]

Through routine assessments, healthcare teams can track disease progression, adjust treatment plans, and provide timely interventions, contributing to improved disease control and quality of life.

Personalized Preventive Strategies

One size does not fit all when it comes to preventive strategies. Personalized approaches to health monitoring allow for tailored interventions based on individual health profiles.

Dr. David L. Katz's work on preventive medicine emphasizes the importance of individualized approaches to disease prevention.[200]

Regular check-ups provide the foundation for assessing individual risk factors and crafting personalized preventive strategies, ranging from dietary modifications to targeted screenings, optimizing the efficacy of preventive efforts.

Encouraging Proactive Lifestyle Changes

Health monitoring serves as a catalyst for proactive lifestyle changes. Dr. Dean Ornish's research on lifestyle medicine highlights the transformative potential of adopting healthier behaviors, such as consuming a whole foods plant based diet, in preventing and managing chronic diseases, especially deadly heart disease and other progressive cardiovascular illnesses.[201]

Regular check-ups provide individuals with tangible metrics, such as cholesterol levels and body mass index (BMI), fostering awareness and motivating proactive changes in diet, exercise, and other lifestyle factors.

In conclusion, the importance of monitoring one's health cannot be overstated. From assessing individual risk factors to detecting silent

---

[199] Eric Topol, "The Patient Will See You Now: The Future of Medicine is in Your Hands," 2015.

[200] David L. Katz, et al., "Preventive Medicine, Integrative Medicine & the Health of the Public," *American Journal of Preventive Medicine*, 2015.

[201] Dean Ornish, et al., "Can lifestyle changes reverse coronary heart disease? The Lifestyle Heart Trial," *The Lancet*, 1990.

conditions and facilitating personalized preventive strategies, routine health check-ups form a cornerstone in the proactive pursuit of optimal health.

KEY DISEASE PREVENTION METHODS

Preventing diseases hinges upon adopting a comprehensive approach that encompasses various evidence-based methods.

In this section, we will explore the key disease prevention methods supported by scientific research and expert insights, providing readers with a robust understanding of proactive health strategies.

Lifestyle Modifications

Dr. David L. Katz, a prominent figure in preventive medicine, emphasizes the transformative potential of lifestyle modifications.[202]

Numerous studies, including those cited by Dr. Katz, highlight the profound impact of lifestyle changes in preventing chronic diseases. From dietary adjustments to regular physical activity, lifestyle modifications play a pivotal role in mitigating risk factors associated with cardiovascular diseases, diabetes, and obesity.

Adopting a plant-based diet, as recommended by Dr. Caldwell B. Esselstyn's research, has been shown to reduce the risk of heart disease and contribute to overall cardiovascular health.[203]

Prudent Vaccination Strategies

Dr. Paul Offit, a renowned vaccine expert, underscores the importance of vaccinations in preventing infectious diseases.[204] The work of Dr. Offit and other vaccine experts highlights the efficacy of vaccination strategies in controlling the spread of certain diseases such as measles, mumps, rubella and smallpox.

---

[202] David L. Katz, et al., "Preventive Medicine, Integrative Medicine & the Health of the Public," *American Journal of Preventive Medicine*, 2015.

[203] Caldwell B. Esselstyn, et al., "A way to reverse CAD?" *Journal of Family Practice*, 2014.

[204] Paul A. Offit, "Vaccinated: One Man's Quest to Defeat the World's Deadliest Diseases," 2007.

While vaccines have likely been instrumental in preventing the spread of a myriad of infectious diseases, they do come with significant risks, including death.

Other illnesses like influenza, the common cold and COVID-19 do not yet respond as well to vaccination strategies since the infectious agents mutate regularly.

Consuming a plant-based diet and regularly supplementing with vitamin C and D3 during winter months tends to have better results than vaccination when it comes to preventing these latter diseases from taking hold.

Screening and Early Detection

The American Cancer Society advocates for routine screenings to facilitate early detection of various cancers.[205] Early detection significantly enhances the chances of successful intervention and treatment.

Regular screenings, such as mammograms and colonoscopies, allow for the identification of abnormalities before they progress to advanced stages. When ionizing radiation is used in the screening process, such as with x-rays and mammograms, it can actually cause cancer, according to the National Cancer Institute[206].

Screenings for breast cancer that do not use radiation are recommended to help detect tumors at an early, more treatable stage, thereby reducing mortality rates from the disease.

The extensive research of Dr. Max Gerson showed that prudent dietary interventions, such as consuming a fully raw plant-based diet and fresh juices, can also be very helpful in preventing cancer and can even assist in reversing the growth of existing tumors.[207]

Genetic Risk Assessment

Geneticists like Dr. Francis Collins emphasize the role of genetic risk assessment in tailoring preventive strategies.[208] Advances in genetic research have paved the way for personalized medicine.

---

[205] American Cancer Society, "Cancer Facts & Figures 2021," 2021.
[206] National Cancer Institute website, retrieved January 2024, URL: https://www.cancer.gov/types/breast/mammograms-fact-sheet
[207] Max Gerson, "A Cancer Therapy: Results of 50 Cases," Totality Books, 1958.

Understanding one's genetic predispositions allows for targeted preventive measures, guiding individuals toward lifestyle modifications and screenings tailored to their unique risk profiles.

Genetic testing for hereditary conditions, such as BRCA mutations associated with breast and ovarian cancers, enables individuals to make better-informed decisions about any proactive health measures they should be taking.

Behavioral Interventions

Behavioral scientists like Dr. Albert Bandura highlight the efficacy of behavioral interventions in promoting health-conscious behaviors.[209] Behavioral interventions focus on modifying habits and promoting positive health behaviors.

Hypnotherapy offers a particularly effective method for behavioral modifications and can serve as a useful intervention technique. From smoking cessation programs to stress management techniques, these interventions contribute to disease prevention by addressing modifiable risk factors.

For example, cognitive-behavioral interventions for smoking cessation, as outlined in research by Dr. Nancy M. Petry, have shown positive outcomes in helping individuals quit tobacco use.[210]

In essence, key disease prevention methods encompass a spectrum of strategies, from lifestyle modifications to vaccinations, early detection, genetic risk assessment, and behavioral interventions. By integrating these evidence-based approaches, individuals can fortify their defenses against a range of diseases, contributing to a proactive and resilient approach to health.

---

[208] Francis S. Collins, "A Vision for the Future of Genomic Research," *Nature*, 2003.

[209] Albert Bandura, "Health promotion from the perspective of social cognitive theory," *Psychology & Health*, 1998.

[210] Nancy M. Petry, "A comprehensive guide to the application of contingency management procedures in clinical settings," *Drug and Alcohol Dependence*, 2000.

EARLY DETECTION OF DISEASE

Early detection forms a linchpin in the paradigm of effective healthcare, offering profound implications for disease management and overall health outcomes.

This section explains how early disease detection works, drawing upon authoritative insights and scientific foundations to underscore its pivotal role in shaping a proactive approach to health.

The Imperative of Timely Intervention

Pioneering work by organizations such as the World Health Organization (WHO) highlights the paramount importance of early detection in reducing disease morbidity and mortality.[211]

Timely intervention, facilitated by early detection, is instrumental in interrupting the natural progression of diseases.

Diseases identified in their nascent stages often present more manageable treatment options, resulting in better prognoses and improved quality of life.

Screening Programs and Diagnostic Technologies

The American Cancer Society and other leading healthcare organizations advocate for structured screening programs to detect cancers early.[212]

Systematic screening programs, coupled with advancements in diagnostic technologies, enhance the capability to identify diseases at their inception.

Modalities such as mammography, colonoscopy, and imaging techniques empower healthcare professionals to pinpoint anomalies before symptomatic manifestations emerge.

Cancer Early Detection Paradigm

Dr. José Baselga's contributions to cancer research emphasize the transformative impact of early detection on cancer outcomes.[213]

---

[211] World Health Organization, "Cancer Control: Knowledge into Action," 2009.
[212] American Cancer Society, "Cancer Facts & Figures 2021," 2021

The cancer early detection paradigm revolves around identifying specific biomarkers and implementing screening measures to detect cancers at a stage when intervention is most effective.

Early detection strategies, exemplified by screenings like Pap smears for cervical cancer, epitomize this approach.

One main caveat for cancer screenings exists, however, because early detection screening techniques that use ionizing radiation like x-rays and mammograms can actually cause cancer, so they should not be used regularly if at all.[214]

Cardiovascular Disease Monitoring

The American Heart Association underscores the importance of regular health check-ups for monitoring cardiovascular health.[215] Cardiovascular diseases, among the leading causes of global morbidity, can often be asymptomatic in their early phases.

Regular health assessments, including blood pressure monitoring and lipid profiling, contribute to the identification of risk factors, enabling interventions to mitigate the progression of cardiovascular diseases.

Furthermore, as the research of Dr. Caldwell B. Esselstyn Jr. has shown, this class of deadly diseases can often be prevented and even reversed by consistently consuming a low-fat plant-based diet.[216]

Type II Diabetes Prevention and Reversal

The American Diabetes Association emphasizes collaborative approaches in the early detection and management of chronic conditions like diabetes.[217]

---

[213] José Baselga, et al., "Phase II Study of Weekly Intravenous Trastuzumab (Herceptin) in Patients With Human Epidermal Growth Factor Receptor 2-Overexpressing Metastatic Breast Cancer," *Journal of Clinical Oncology*, 2004.

[214] Miglioretti DL, Lange J, van den Broek JJ, Lee CI, van Ravesteyn NT, Ritley D, Kerlikowske K, Fenton JJ, Melnikow J, de Koning HJ, Hubbard RA. "Radiation-Induced Breast Cancer Incidence and Mortality From Digital Mammography Screening: A Modeling Study", *Ann. Internal Medicine*, 2016.

[215] American Heart Association, "Heart Disease and Stroke Statistics—2021 Update," 2021.

[216] Caldwell B. Esselstyn Jr., "Prevent and Reverse Heart Disease: The Revolutionary, Scientifically Proven, Nutrition-Based Cure," Avery, 2007.

Type II diabetes has been shown to respond well to weight loss programs and can often be managed with dietary interventions including consuming a raw plant-based diet.

Still, it is important to note that individual responses to dietary changes can vary, and the total reversal of type 2 diabetes may not be universal for all individuals.

The American Diabetes Association (ADA) acknowledges that weight loss and increased physical activity, which may be facilitated by a plant-based diet, can improve insulin sensitivity and glycemic control. They also emphasize that individualized nutrition plans should be developed with healthcare providers.

Furthermore, some research studies have suggested positive outcomes in terms of glycemic control and insulin sensitivity with plant-based diets.[218] In particular, diets that prioritize whole grains, vegetables, fruits, and legumes while excluding animal products have been shown to enhance blood glucose levels, manage body weight, regulate plasma lipid concentrations, and control blood pressure.

These healthier dietary patterns also play a significant role in mitigating the risk of cardiovascular and microvascular complications. With that noted, practical factors such as education, ensuring nutritional adequacy, and making necessary medication adjustments can contribute to the success of individuals managing type II diabetes with a plant-based diet.

Detecting and Preventing Obesity

Obesity, a multifaceted health concern, is now thought of as a chronic disease that demands early detection and proactive interventions. The American Heart Association emphasizes the significance of individualized approaches to obesity prevention and early intervention.[219]

---

[217] American Diabetes Association, "Standards of Medical Care in Diabetes—2021," 2021.

[218] Jardine MA, Kahleova H, Levin SM, Ali Z, Trapp CB, Barnard ND. "Perspective: Plant-Based Eating Pattern for Type 2 Diabetes Prevention and Treatment: Efficacy, Mechanisms, and Practical Considerations." *Advanced Nutrition*, 2021.

[219] Jensen, M. D., et al., "2013 AHA/ACC/TOS Guideline for the Management of Overweight and Obesity in Adults," *Circulation*, 2014.

Regular health check-ups, including monitoring metabolic parameters, contribute to early detection and tailored management strategies. Healthcare professionals can integrate personalized assessments into routine check-ups, incorporating measurements like body mass index (BMI), waist circumference, and biomarkers associated with metabolic health.

Basically, early identification enables timely interventions when it comes to combatting obesity. On the bright side, the integration of a low-fat plant-based diet and hypnotherapy emerges as a promising strategy in the prevention and treatment of obesity, combining nutritional efficacy with psychological support.

Numerous studies, including research by Dr. Neal Barnard and colleagues, underscore the effectiveness of plant-based diets in weight management.[220] The emphasis on whole grains, fruits, vegetables, and legumes aligns with nutritional principles linked to reduced obesity risk.

Encouraging obese individuals to adopt a low-fat plant-centric dietary approach involves education on meal planning, nutrient balance, and addressing concerns related to dietary changes. Research shows that low-fat plant-based diets can contribute substantially to weight loss and maintenance.[221]

Furthermore, hypnotherapy, as explored in studies by Dr. Susan Hepburn and Dr. Jean Kristeller, offers a complementary approach to traditional weight management strategies.[222] By targeting behavioral patterns and promoting mindful eating, hypnotherapy addresses the psychological aspects of obesity.

Integrating hypnotherapy into obesity prevention involves personalized sessions that address emotional triggers, stress-related eating, and the

---

[220] Barnard, N. D., et al., "A Systematic Review and Meta-Analysis of Changes in Body Weight in Clinical Trials of Vegetarian Diets," *Journal of the Academy of Nutrition and Dietetics*, 2015.

[221] Turner-McGrievy, G. M., et al., "Comparing the Dietary Guidelines for Americans, Vegetarian Diets and the Mediterranean Diet for Weight Loss," *Nutrients*, 2015.

[222] Hepburn, S. R., "Cognitive-Behavioral Hypnotherapy in the Treatment of Emotional and Behavioral Symptoms of Menopause," *Menopause: The Journal of The North American Menopause Society*, 2012.

establishment of positive behavioral habits. Hypnotherapy has demonstrated efficacy in supporting long-term weight management.[223]

In conclusion, the early detection and prevention of obesity necessitate a holistic strategy that encompasses nutritional guidance, psychological support, and personalized monitoring.

The integration of a plant-based diet and hypnotherapy stands as a scientifically grounded approach, providing individuals with effective tools to address obesity from both physiological and psychological perspectives.

The Helpful Role of Genetic Screening

Geneticists and healthcare experts, including Dr. Francis Collins, emphasize the role of genetic screening in identifying hereditary conditions early.[224]

Genetic screening offers a unique avenue for early detection, particularly for conditions with a hereditary component.

Identifying genetic markers associated with diseases allows for proactive measures and tailored interventions based on individual risk profiles.

Preventive Measures Informed by Early Detection

Research by Dr. Russell Harris elucidates the critical link between early detection and the formulation of preventive measures.[225]

Early detection not only enables timely treatment but also informs the implementation of preventive strategies. For instance, identifying precancerous lesions through screenings can prompt interventions to prevent the development of full-blown cancers.

In essence, early detection serves as a linchpin in the healthcare continuum, offering a proactive stance against the progression of diseases. From structured screening programs to leveraging cutting-edge diagnostic

---

[223] Kristeller, J. L., et al., "Mindfulness Meditation, Well-Being, and Eating: Applying Positive Psychology to Improve Attitudes toward Food and Eating," Mindfulness, 2013.

[224] Francis S. Collins, "A Vision for the Future of Genomic Research," *Nature*, 2003.

[225] Russell P. Harris, et al., "Screening for colorectal cancer: systematic review," *JAMA*, 2008.

technologies, the science of early detection stands as a beacon for improved health outcomes and a cornerstone of comprehensive healthcare strategies.

COLLABORATING WITH HEALTHCARE PROFESSIONALS

The synergy between individuals and healthcare professionals is the linchpin for optimal health, fostering a proactive and informed approach to well-being.

In this section, we will explore the profound significance of collaborative relationships between individuals and healthcare professionals, drawing upon authoritative insights and scientific foundations to elucidate the transformative impact on health outcomes.

In particular, we will look at the transformative impact on health outcomes through patient-centered care, regular health assessments, chronic disease management, telehealth technologies, genetic counseling, and health education.

Patient-Centered Care

The Institute of Medicine underscores the pivotal role of patient-centered care in fostering collaborative relationships between individuals and healthcare professionals.[226]

Patient-centered care places individuals at the forefront of their healthcare process, involving them as active participants in decision-making so that suitable care choices can be made.

This approach, supported by research in healthcare delivery, empowers individuals to play a proactive role in shaping their health trajectories.

Regular Health Assessments and Preventive Care

The Centers for Disease Control and Prevention (CDC) advocates for regular health assessments to facilitate preventive care.[227]

---

[226] Institute of Medicine, "Crossing the Quality Chasm: A New Health System for the 21st Century," 2001.
[227] Centers for Disease Control and Prevention, "The Power of Prevention: Chronic Disease... The Public Health Challenge of the 21st Century," 2009.

Regular health assessments, conducted in collaboration with healthcare professionals, serve as a linchpin for preventive care strategies.

Through regular disease screenings that do not include ionizing radiation, taking certain highly-effective vaccinations, prudent behavioral adjustments, and lifestyle counseling, individuals can work alongside healthcare providers to mitigate health risk factors.

They can also adopt proactive health-promoting measures like consuming a low-fat plant-based diet as a well-tested form of effective preventative care.

Chronic Disease Management

Chronic diseases can necessitate ongoing management, so forging constructive collaborative relationships between individuals and healthcare professionals are critical for successful treatment.

Shared decision-making, personalized treatment plans, and continuous monitoring contribute to effective chronic disease management.

Furthermore, certain chronic diseases typically respond well to plant-based dietary interventions. These include cardiovascular disease, obesity, cancers and diabetes.[228]

Using Telehealth Technologies

Dr. Ateev Mehrotra's research on telehealth underscores its potential in fostering collaborative healthcare delivery.[229]

Telehealth technologies offer innovative avenues for collaboration, enabling individuals to connect with healthcare professionals remotely.

Virtual consultations, remote monitoring, and telemedicine contribute to accessible and timely healthcare interventions.

Genetic Counseling and Personalized Medicine

Genetic counselors, in collaboration with healthcare providers, play a key

---

[228] American Diabetes Association, "Standards of Medical Care in Diabetes—2021," 2021.
[229] Ateev Mehrotra, et al., "The Impact of the COVID-19 Pandemic on Outpatient Visits: A Rebound Emerges," *The Commonwealth Fund*, 2020.

role in guiding individuals through genetic risk assessments.[230] In the realm of personalized medicine, genetic counseling becomes integral.

Collaborative efforts between individuals, genetic counselors, and healthcare professionals allow for more informed decision-making based on genetic predispositions.

This process can contribute substantially to tailoring effective preventive healthcare strategies.

Health Education and Empowerment

Health educators, in collaboration with healthcare professionals, contribute to empowering individuals through education and awareness.[231]

Health education is a vital component of collaborative care, providing individuals with the knowledge and tools to make informed decisions about their health.

Educational initiatives on nutrition, physical activity, and preventive measures enhance health literacy and foster proactive health behaviors.

Conclusion

In conclusion, collaborative relationships between individuals and healthcare professionals form a symbiotic alliance, driving a proactive and informed approach to health.

From patient-centered care principles to leveraging telehealth technologies and embracing personalized medicine, collaboration emerges as a catalyst for transformative healthcare experiences.

---

[230] National Society of Genetic Counselors, "About Genetic Counselors," 2021.
[231] Society for Public Health Education, "What is Health Education?" 2021.

CHAPTER 9: LIFELONG LEARNING AND INTELLECTUAL VITALITY

INTRODUCTION

In the pursuit of longevity and overall well-being, our study now extends beyond dietary considerations and physical health into the realm of intellectual vitality. Chapter 9 thus explores the significance of lifelong learning as a key component of a holistic approach to health with three integral sections that illuminate the connection between intellectual stimulation and longevity.

Scientific understanding supports the notion that cognitive engagement plays a pivotal role in maintaining brain health throughout the lifespan. Respected authorities in neuroscience, such as Dr. Sandra Bond Chapman and Dr. Michael Merzenich, have extensively explored the concept of neuroplasticity—the brain's remarkable ability to adapt and grow in response to stimuli.[232] [233] The first section of this chapter will elucidate the strategies and activities that promote mental acuity, emphasizing the role of challenging cognitive tasks and novel experiences.

The pursuit of knowledge is not confined to any specific age; instead, it thrives in a lifelong commitment to learning. Drawing on the expertise of educational psychologists like Dr. Carol S. Dweck, the second section of this chapter advocates for a growth mindset—an approach that perceives challenges as opportunities for learning and embraces the belief in one's capacity for intellectual development.[234] Practical insights and evidence-based recommendations illuminate the path to continuous learning.

The detailed connection between intellectual stimulation and overall well-being is a theme explored by renowned researchers such as Dr. Laura L.

---

[232] Chapman, S. B., et al., "Neural Mechanisms of Brain Plasticity with Cognitive Training in Healthy Adults," *Frontiers in Aging Neuroscience,* 2015.
[233] Merzenich, M. M., et al., "Neural Plasticity-Based Training Approaches in Aphasia Rehabilitation: Theoretic Background and Clinical Realities," *Aphasiology,* 2014.
[234] Dweck, C. S., "Mindset: The New Psychology of Success," *Random House,* 2006.

Carstensen. Scientific evidence suggests that sustained mental engagement positively influences emotional health and contributes to a sense of purpose and fulfillment.[235] The final section of this chapter unpacks the mechanisms through which intellectual pursuits enhance the quality of life, emphasizing the close relationship between cognitive vitality and holistic well-being.

In a contemporary twist, this chapter also explores the role of stimulating and strategic video games as tools for mental engagement. Studies by experts like Dr. Daphne Bavelier and Dr. Adam Gazzaley shed light on how such video games can serve as effective instruments for cognitive stimulation.[236] [237] Practical examples and insights highlight the potential benefits of integrating strategic gaming into a lifelong learning strategy.

As you embark on the exploration of intellectual vitality and its profound implications for longevity, let this chapter serve as your guide to fostering a curious, agile, and ever-evolving mind well into your golden years.

STIMULATING THE MIND FOR LONGEVITY

In the pursuit of cognitive longevity, the scientific exploration of strategies to stimulate the mind unveils a multifaceted approach encompassing diverse activities and experiences.

This section goes into the detailed mechanisms behind stimulating the mind for enhanced cognitive vitality, with a contemporary focus on the role of stimulating and strategic video games.

Cognitive Engagement and Neuroplasticity

The foundation of stimulating the mind lies in the profound concept of neuroplasticity— the brain's remarkable ability to adapt and reorganize itself in response to external stimuli.

---

[235] Carstensen, L. L., "The Influence of a Sense of Time on Human Development," *Science,* 2006.

[236] Bavelier, D., et al., "Cognitive Neuroscience: Training the Brain: Fact and Fiction," *Psychological Science in the Public Interest,* 2013.

[237] Gazzaley, A., et al., "Neuroplasticity: A Double-Edged Sword," *Brain,* 2018.

Esteemed neuroscientists such as Dr. Sandra Bond Chapman and Dr. Michael Merzenich have extensively researched the neural mechanisms underpinning cognitive engagement.[238] [239] Engaging in challenging cognitive tasks, problem-solving activities, and exposure to novel experiences fosters the rewiring of neural circuits, contributing to improved cognitive function.

Strategic Video Games and Cognitive Stimulation

In the contemporary world of cognitive enhancement, strategic video games emerge as intriguing tools for mental stimulation. Research led by experts such as Dr. Daphne Bavelier and Dr. Adam Gazzaley has elucidated the cognitive benefits of playing these games. [240] [241]

These games often demand strategic thinking, rapid decision-making, and multitasking, engaging various cognitive functions. For instance, action games have been linked to improvements in attention, visual processing, and spatial skills, showcasing the potential of digital platforms in contributing to cognitive resilience.

The Role of Dopaminergic Systems

Scientific investigations into the effects of stimulating activities on cognitive longevity highlight the involvement of dopaminergic systems in the brain.

Dopamine, a neurotransmitter associated with reward and pleasure, plays an important role in modulating cognitive functions.

Activities that induce a sense of challenge and achievement, such as solving complex puzzles or playing video games, can trigger dopamine release, promoting a positive feedback loop for sustained cognitive engagement.

---

[238] Chapman, S. B., et al., "Neural Mechanisms of Brain Plasticity with Cognitive Training in Healthy Adults," *Frontiers in Aging Neuroscience,* 2015.

[239] Merzenich, M. M., et al., "Neural Plasticity-Based Training Approaches in Aphasia Rehabilitation: Theoretic Background and Clinical Realities," *Aphasiology,* 2014.

[240] Bavelier, D., et al., "Cognitive Neuroscience: Training the Brain: Fact and Fiction," *Psychological Science in the Public Interest,* 2013.

[241] Gazzaley, A., et al., "Neuroplasticity: A Double-Edged Sword," *Brain,* 2018.

Practical Applications in Lifelong Learning

Integrating stimulating activities, including strategic video games, into a lifelong learning framework becomes an actionable strategy for promoting cognitive vitality.

Beyond traditional approaches, harnessing the interactive and dynamic nature of digital platforms offers individuals diverse avenues for continuous mental engagement.

As you start to unravel the details of stimulating the mind for longevity, the integration of tools like strategic video games into cognitive enhancement practices emerges as a contemporary and scientifically grounded dimension, showcasing the evolving process of lifelong learning.

ENGAGING IN CONTINUOUS LEARNING AND GROWTH

The pursuit of cognitive longevity unfolds not merely as a static state but as an ongoing process marked by continuous learning and growth.

This section explores the scientific understanding of the profound benefits derived from a commitment to perpetual learning, with a contemporary lens on how challenging cognitive activities like playing strategic video games can contribute to this dynamic process.

Neurobiological Foundations of Continuous Learning

At the core of engaging in continuous learning is the neurobiological principle of synaptic plasticity—the ability of synapses to strengthen or weaken over time. Esteemed neuroscientists such as Dr. Carol S. Dweck and Dr. Michael Merzenich have explored the neurobiological foundations of growth mindset and continuous learning. [242] [243]

Embracing challenges and seeking new knowledge triggers neural adaptations, fostering cognitive flexibility and resilience.

---

[242] Dweck, C. S., "Mindset: The New Psychology of Success," *Random House,* 2006.
[243] Merzenich, M. M., et al., "Neural Plasticity-Based Training Approaches in Aphasia Rehabilitation: Theoretic Background and Clinical Realities," *Aphasiology,* 2014.

The Evolutionary Advantage of a Growth Mindset

The concept of a growth mindset, as championed by Dr. Dweck, posits that viewing challenges as opportunities for learning and embracing a belief in one's capacity for intellectual development promotes cognitive growth.[244]

This adaptive mindset aligns with the evolutionary advantage conferred by a brain that remains plastic, agile, and receptive to novel stimuli—an asset in navigating an ever-changing environment.

Strategic Video Games as Tools for Continuous Learning

In the digital age, strategic video games emerge as compelling instruments for continuous learning. Research by experts such as Dr. Daphne Bavelier and Dr. Adam Gazzaley has demonstrated that these games often require the mastery of new skills and the adaptation to evolving challenges. [245] [246]

The dynamic nature of these games mirrors the ongoing learning process, demanding players to continuously engage in problem-solving, strategic thinking, and the acquisition of new knowledge.

Realizing Cognitive Growth Through Digital Platforms

As individuals tread the path of continuous learning and growth as they age, the integration of cognitive tools like strategic video games into life can become a contemporary scientifically-grounded strategy for mental stimulation.

These games offer a unique platform for users to acquire and apply new knowledge, honing cognitive skills in an interactive and engaging manner. They can also offer social experiences that aging people can use to replace more traditional interaction activities as their mobility and social circle diminishes over time.

This exploration of engaging in continuous learning illuminates the relationship between neurobiological adaptability, growth mindset, and the

---

[244] Dweck, C. S., "Mindset: The New Psychology of Success," *Random House,* 2006.
[245] Bavelier, D., et al., "Cognitive Neuroscience: Training the Brain: Fact and Fiction," *Psychological Science in the Public Interest,* 2013.
[246] Gazzaley, A., et al. , "Neuroplasticity: A Double-Edged Sword," *Brain,* 2018.

modern avenues, such as strategic video games, through which individuals can start the process of furthering their perpetual cognitive evolution.

INTELLECTUAL STIMULATION AND WELL-BEING

The close connection between intellectual stimulation and overall well-being emerges as a cornerstone in the pursuit of cognitive longevity.

This section elucidates the scientific underpinnings of how engaging in intellectually stimulating activities, including puzzle solving and strategic video games, can significantly contribute to promoting well-being and, by extension, longevity.

Cognitive Engagement and Emotional Well-Being

Scientific investigations spearheaded by researchers like Dr. Laura L. Carstensen reveal a compelling link between sustained cognitive engagement and emotional well-being.[247]

Engaging in intellectually stimulating activities not only exercises the brain but also triggers the release of neurotransmitters associated with pleasure and reward. This relationship fosters a positive emotional state, contributing to an overall sense of well-being.

Strategic Video Games and Emotional Resilience

In the digital era, strategic video games offer a unique avenue for intellectual stimulation that extends beyond mere entertainment. Studies conducted by experts such as Dr. Daphne Bavelier and Dr. Adam Gazzaley shed light on the cognitive benefits of playing these games. [248] [249]

By challenging cognitive faculties and demanding strategic thinking, these games promote a state of "flow," wherein individuals experience heightened focus and a sense of accomplishment—factors needed for emotional resilience.

---

[247] Carstensen, L. L., "The Influence of a Sense of Time on Human Development," *Science*, 2006.

[248] Bavelier, D., et al., "Cognitive Neuroscience: Training the Brain: Fact and Fiction," *Psychological Science in the Public Interest*, 2013.

[249] Gazzaley, A., et al., "Neuroplasticity: A Double-Edged Sword," *Brain*, 2018.

Enhancing Quality of Life Through Intellectual Pursuits

The connection between intellectual pursuits and an enhanced quality of life is underscored by the positive impact of cognitive engagement on various domains.

From improved stress management to the cultivation of a sense of purpose, intellectual stimulation contributes to a holistic state of well-being.

By incorporating intellectually stimulating activities like solving puzzles, doing brain teasers, and playing strategic video games into your daily routine, you can actively participate in the cultivation of these positive outcomes.

Nurturing Cognitive Health for Longevity

As you start to understand the link between intellectual stimulation and well-being, strategic video games emerge as contemporary tools that align with the principles of neuroplasticity and emotional resilience.

The integration of such activities into a comprehensive approach to lifelong learning can offer a dynamic solution for nurturing cognitive health and promoting longevity.

CHAPTER 10: CULTIVATING A POSITIVE MINDSET

INTRODUCTION

In the study of longevity, your mental environment plays a pivotal role. This chapter focuses on cultivating a positive mindset and explores the profound impact of positive mental states on overall well-being and longevity.

Rooted in scientific understanding, this chapter unfolds the multifaceted dimensions of positivity, affirmations, optimism, and the interconnectedness of mind and body. As you examine the scientific literature on this fascinating topic, you will uncover the compelling evidence supporting the transformative power of a positive mindset.

Scientific research, including studies by Dr. Barbara L. Fredrickson and Dr. Sonja Lyubomirsky, has underscored the far-reaching benefits of cultivating a positive mindset. [250] [251] Positivity not only enhances emotional well-being but also contributes to physical health, fostering resilience against stress and promoting cardiovascular health.

As we then delve into the realm of cognitive science, the section on affirmations and prayer draws insights from studies by Dr. Joanne V. Wood and Dr. Andrew Newberg. [252] [253] These practices, when approached with a positive mindset, exhibit neurobiological effects, influencing areas of the brain associated with emotional regulation and resilience.

---

[250] Fredrickson, B. L., "The Role of Positive Emotions in Positive Psychology: The Broaden-and-Build Theory of Positive Emotions," *American Psychologist,* 2001.

[251] Lyubomirsky, S., et al., "Pursuing Happiness: The Architecture of Sustainable Change," *Review of General Psychology,* 2005.

[252] Wood, J. V., et al., "Positive Self-Statements: Power for Some, Peril for Others," *Psychological Science,* 2009.

[253] Newberg, A., et al., "The Measurement of Regional Cerebral Blood Flow During Glossolalia: A Preliminary SPECT Study," *Psychiatry Research: Neuroimaging,* 2001.

This chapter will next explore the realms of optimism and gratitude, referencing the works of Dr. Martin E. P. Seligman and Dr. Robert A. Emmons.[254] [255] Their research shows that optimism acts as a psychological buffer against adversity, while gratitude practices contribute to increased life satisfaction and well-being.

Scientific endeavors by researchers like Dr. Herbert Benson have also illuminated the detailed connection between the mind and body. [256] Understanding how positive mental states influence physiological processes unveils a pathway to harnessing this mind-body connection for optimal health and longevity.

Drawing from social psychology and epidemiology, the final section of this chapter references studies by Dr. Nicholas A. Christakis and Dr. James H. Fowler.[257] [258] Surrounding oneself with positive social circles not only enhances individual well-being but also exhibits a ripple effect, influencing the health and longevity of the broader community.

As you embark on the path of cultivating a positive mindset, let each section of this chapter unfold as a testament to the scientific underpinnings of positivity and its profound implications for a longer and healthier life.

THE POWER OF POSITIVITY

At the nexus of psychology and health science lays the compelling exploration of the power of cultivating positivity when it comes to longevity. Researchers such as Dr. Barbara L. Fredrickson have studied the complex mechanisms by which positive emotions wield influence over our mental and physical well-being.[259]

---

[254] Seligman, M. E. P. "Learned Optimism: How to Change Your Mind and Your Life," *Vintage,* 2006.

[255] Emmons, R. A., et al., "Counting Blessings Versus Burdens: An Experimental Investigation of Gratitude and Subjective Well-Being in Daily Life," *Journal of Personality and Social Psychology,* 2003.

[256] Benson, H., et al., "The Relaxation Response," *Psychiatry,* 1975.

[257] Christakis, N. A., & Fowler, J. H., "The Collective Dynamics of Smoking in a Large Social Network," *New England Journal of Medicine,* 2008.

[258] Fowler, J. H., & Christakis, N. A., "Dynamic Spread of Happiness in a Large Social Network: Longitudinal Analysis over 20 Years in the Framingham Heart Study," *British Medical Journal,* 2008.

Fredrickson's Broaden-and-Build Theory proposes that positive emotions broaden an individual's thought-action repertoire, fostering resilience and adaptability.

This not only enhances psychological well-being but also contributes to the physical health of an individual. Studies conducted on the effects of positive emotions, as reviewed by Fredrickson, consistently highlight their role in buffering against stress, promoting cardiovascular health, and bolstering immune function.[260]

Positivity, as a psychological state, acts as a protective factor, mitigating the impact of stressors on mental health. Notably, positive emotions are associated with decreased levels of cortisol, the stress hormone, and contribute to an individual's emotional resilience.[261]

Moreover, the cardiovascular benefits of positivity extend beyond stress reduction. Positive emotions have been linked to improved heart health, with studies showing a lower risk of cardiovascular diseases in individuals characterized by a positive emotional outlook. [262]

The Profound Impact of Positivity on Well-Being

Within the scientific exploration of cultivating a positive mindset, the profound impact of positivity on well-being emerges as a multifaceted aspect deeply rooted in psychological research.

As you explore the scientific terrain of the profound impact of positivity on well-being and longevity, it should become increasingly evident that positivity transcends the realms of mere optimism. It is a dynamic force closely linked to mental resilience, adaptive coping mechanisms, and the cultivation of enduring personal resources—all of which contribute significantly to a longer and healthier life.

Furthermore, fostering a positive mindset is not merely a subjective endeavor but a scientifically supported strategy for promoting mental and physical health. Embracing positivity, as substantiated by empirical

---

[259] Fredrickson, B. L., "The Role of Positive Emotions in Positive Psychology: The Broaden-and-Build Theory of Positive Emotions," *American Psychologist,* 2001.
[260] Fredrickson, B. L., ibid.
[261] Fredrickson, B. L., ibid.
[262] Fredrickson, B. L., ibid.

evidence, emerges as a potent tool for cultivating a foundation of well-being that supports longevity.

Drawing from the extensive works of notable figures in positive psychology, such as Dr. Martin E. P. Seligman and Dr. Barbara L. Fredrickson, the rest of this section seeks to unravel the complex dynamics of positivity, offering empirical evidence of its far-reaching implications for mental states and longevity. [263] [264]

Positivity and Mental Resilience

Dr. Martin E. P. Seligman, a pioneer in positive psychology, has extensively studied the concept of positivity and its implications for mental health. At its core, positivity is not merely about an optimistic outlook; it encompasses a broader array of positive emotions and experiences.

Seligman's seminal work highlights positivity as a vital element contributing to mental resilience, providing individuals with the cognitive tools to navigate challenges with greater efficacy.

Empirical studies have underscored the association between positivity and mental well-being. Individuals fostering a positive mindset are more adept at coping with stress, exhibit lower levels of depression and anxiety, and generally report higher life satisfaction.[265]

This detailed interaction between positive emotions and mental resilience positions positivity as a cornerstone in the cultivation of a robust and enduring mental state.

The Broaden-and-Build Theory

Dr. Barbara L. Fredrickson's renowned Broaden-and-Build Theory further deepens our understanding of positivity's impact. According to this theory, positive emotions broaden an individual's momentary thought-action repertoire, fostering creativity and open-mindedness.[266]

---

[263] Seligman, M. E. P., "Learned Optimism: How to Change Your Mind and Your Life," Vintage, 2006.
[264] Fredrickson, B. L., "The Role of Positive Emotions in Positive Psychology: The Broaden-and-Build Theory of Positive Emotions," *American Psychologist,* 2001.
[265] Seligman, M. E. P., ibid.
[266] Fredrickson, B. L., ibid.

Over time, this broadening effect builds enduring personal resources, contributing to increased psychological resilience and overall well-being. Further research on Fredrickson's theory has demonstrated that the experience of positive emotions, even in fleeting moments, holds the potential to enhance an individual's resilience and adaptive capacities.

From fostering social connections to promoting physical health, positivity becomes a catalyst for building enduring personal resources that transcend the immediate emotional experience.

THE VALUE OF AFFIRMATIONS AND PRAYER

In the realm of mental practices that influence well-being, exploring the value of affirmations and prayer unveils cognitive and neurobiological elements.

This section offers insight into scientific inquiries on the topic, citing authorities like Dr. Joanne V. Wood and Dr. Andrew Newberg, to examine the profound impact of these practices on mental states and their potential implications for longevity. [267] [268]

Cognitive Science and Affirmations

Affirmations, positive statements focused on one's strengths or desired outcomes, have garnered attention in cognitive science. Research led by Dr. Joanne V. Wood emphasizes the role of self-affirmation in mitigating the impact of stressors on individuals' mental well-being. [269]

The cognitive mechanisms at play involve reinforcing positive self-identity, enhancing self-integrity, and creating a buffer against the psychological toll of stress.

---

[267] Wood, J. V., et al., "Positive Self-Statements: Power for Some, Peril for Others," *Psychological Science,* 2009.

[268] Newberg, A., et al., "The Measurement of Regional Cerebral Blood Flow During Glossolalia: A Preliminary SPECT Study," *Psychiatry Research: Neuroimaging,* 2001.

[269] Wood, J. V., et al., ibid.

Studies in cognitive psychology highlight that engaging in affirmations can contribute to improved problem-solving skills and increased resilience by shaping a mindset conducive to positive mental states. [270]

Neurobiological Insights into Prayer

The intersection of neurobiology and spirituality is navigated through the exploration of prayer. Dr. Andrew Newberg's investigations into the neuroscientific aspects of religious and spiritual practices provide a lens through which the value of prayer can be understood.[271]

Neuroimaging studies reveal that prayer and other forms of religious engagement activate specific brain regions associated with positive emotions and a sense of connection.

Newberg's work suggests that prayer may induce neuroplastic changes, potentially enhancing emotional regulation and stress resilience. The neurobiological responses to prayer underscore its potential role in fostering a positive mindset and contributing to mental well-being.

As you learn about the value of affirmations and prayer, it may become evident to you that these practices are not confined to the realms of faith or personal empowerment but extend their influence into the fabric of mental and emotional resilience.

Grounded in scientific exploration, affirmations and prayer emerge as tools with the potential to sculpt a positive mindset, offering a pathway towards greater well-being and longevity.

FOSTERING OPTIMISM AND GRATITUDE

Within the scientific exploration of cultivating a positive mindset, the facets of fostering optimism and gratitude emerge as integral components deeply rooted in psychological and well-being research.

Drawing from the works of Dr. Martin E. P. Seligman and Dr. Robert A. Emmons, this section unravels the complex dynamics of optimism and gratitude, elucidating their profound impact on mental states and longevity. [272] [273]

---

[270] Wood, J. V., et al., ibid.
[271] Newberg, A., et al., ibid.

Optimism as a Psychological Resilience Tool

Dr. Martin E. P. Seligman, a pioneer in positive psychology, has extensively studied the concept of optimism and its implications for mental health. Optimism, characterized by a positive outlook on future outcomes, is recognized as a psychological resilience tool that can buffer against the adverse effects of stress and adversity.[274]

Studies in positive psychology have demonstrated that cultivating optimism is associated with lower levels of depression, increased life satisfaction, and enhanced overall well-being. Optimistic individuals exhibit a greater capacity to cope with life's challenges, fostering a mental state conducive to longevity. [275]

Gratitude's Impact on Well-Being

Delving into the realm of gratitude, Dr. Robert A. Emmons' research has provided valuable insights into its impact on well-being. Gratitude, defined as a positive emotional response to kindness or generosity, has been linked to a myriad of psychological and physical health benefits. [276]

Scientific investigations reveal that practicing gratitude is associated with increased levels of positive emotions, improved sleep quality, and reduced symptoms of depression and anxiety. Moreover, gratitude has been found to contribute to enhanced cardiovascular health, emphasizing its role in fostering a holistic state of well-being. [277]

As you navigate the science of fostering optimism and gratitude, it should become more and more evident that these mental practices transcend mere positive thinking. They are empirically substantiated tools that shape cognitive perspectives and emotional experiences and are woven into the fabric of a positive mindset conducive to a longer and healthier life.

---

[272] Seligman, M. E. P., "Learned Optimism: How to Change Your Mind and Your Life," *Vintage*, 2006.

[273] Emmons, R. A., et al., "Counting Blessings Versus Burdens: An Experimental Investigation of Gratitude and Subjective Well-Being in Daily Life," *Journal of Personality and Social Psychology,* 2003.

[274] Seligman, M. E. P., ibid.

[275] Seligman, M. E. P., ibid.

[276] Emmons, R. A., et al., ibid.

[277] Emmons, R. A., et al., ibid.

HARNESSING THE MIND-BODY CONNECTION FOR HEALTH

Exploring the complex web of connections between mental states and physical well-being unravels a profound insight into the mind-body connection.

This section delves into studies on the topic, drawing from the works of Dr. Herbert Benson and Dr. Esther M. Sternberg, to explain the ways in which the mind influences the body and, consequently, your overall health. [278] [279]

Mind-Body Medicine

Dr. Herbert Benson, a trailblazer in mind-body medicine, has conducted seminal research on the physiological impacts of mental practices. His work emphasizes the role of the mind in eliciting the relaxation response, a state counteracting the stress response and promoting physical well-being.[280]

Studies on mind-body interventions, such as meditation and deep breathing, have revealed their potential to modulate the autonomic nervous system, reduce inflammation, and enhance immune function. These physiological changes underscore the tangible impact of mental practices on the body's health.[281]

The Interplay of Mind and Immune System

The intersection of psychology, neuroscience, and immunology is explored through the field of psychoneuroimmunology, and Dr. Esther M. Sternberg's contributions have been instrumental in unraveling the complex interactions between the mind and the immune system.[282]

Research in psychoneuroimmunology highlights how mental states, including stress and positive emotions, can influence immune function. Chronic stress, for instance, has been linked to immunosuppression, while

---

[278] Benson, H., et al., "The Relaxation Response," *Psychiatry,* 1975.
[279] Sternberg, E. M., "Neural Regulation of Innate Immunity: A Coordinate Action of Brain and Adaptive Autonomic Responses," *Molecular Psychiatry,* 2006.
[280] Benson, H., et al., ibid.
[281] Benson, H., et al., ibid.
[282] Sternberg, E. M., ibid.

positive emotions can enhance immune responses. These findings underscore the dynamic interplay between mental well-being and the body's ability to defend against illness. [283]

As we navigate the scientific terrain of "Harnessing the Mind-Body Connection for Health," it becomes apparent that the mind is not a passive observer but an active participant in shaping our physical health. Cultivating a positive mindset, as substantiated by scientific inquiry, emerges as a pivotal aspect of promoting overall health and longevity.

BEING KIND ENHANCES MOOD AND CONSCIENCE

In the interplay between mind and body, the choices we make regarding our diet and the harm it can cause to other living beings can carry profound implications not only for physical health but also for mental well-being.

Delving into the ethical dimensions of dietary decisions, particularly the choice to adopt a kinder plant-based diet and thereby avoid directly causing harm to animals, sheds light on the causal relationship between kinder lifestyle choices and more positive psychological states.

The Advantage of an Ethical Diet for Mind and Body

Scientific literature, including studies such as those conducted by Dr. Dean Ornish and Dr. Neal D. Barnard, consistently underscores the health benefits of plant-based diets.

You have already read that plant-based dieters tend to run a reduced risk of chronic diseases. Improved cardiovascular health, a better body mass index, and enhanced overall well-being are also among the physiological advantages associated with plant-centric eating patterns. [284] [285]

However, the benefits extend beyond the physical realm. Adopting a plant-based diet, rooted in the principle of not causing harm to animals, aligns

---

[283] Sternberg, E. M., ibid.

[284] Ornish, D., et al., "Can Lifestyle Changes Reverse Coronary Heart Disease? The Lifestyle Heart Trial," *The Lancet*, 1998.

[285] Barnard, N. D., et al., "A Systematic Review and Meta-Analysis of Changes in Body Weight in Clinical Trials of Vegetarian Diets," *Journal of the Academy of Nutrition and Dietetics*, 2009.

with the virtue of kindness and other ethical considerations that can positively influence mental states.

Research has suggested a correlation between ethical dietary choices and enhanced mood and emotional well-being. The conscious decision to avoid contributing to the harm of sentient beings fosters a sense of alignment with one's values, contributing to a more positive and harmonious psychological state.

Psychological Impact of Ethical Eating

The interconnectedness of dietary choices and psychological well-being is evident in the psychological impact of ethical eating. Studies have explored the emotional benefits of adopting ethical dietary practices, emphasizing the positive effects on mood, empathy, and a heightened sense of moral alignment.[286]

In fact, choosing a plant-based diet, motivated by a commitment to being kind to other living beings can serve as a powerful catalyst for a positive shift in one's psychological landscape. The alignment of dietary choices with ethical values not only contributes to physical health but also nurtures a heightened awareness of the interconnectedness of our actions and their impact on the well-being of other animals.

Overall, the ethical dimensions of dietary choices emerge as a transformative force for positivity in one's life. Choosing a plant-based lifestyle not only fosters physical health but also aligns with ethical considerations, paving the way for an enhanced mood, a clear conscience, and a deeper connection with the broader network of life.

SURROUND YOURSELF WITH POSITIVE PEOPLE

When cultivating a positive mindset, your social fabric plays a pivotal role in shaping your personal well-being. This section explores scientific insights, drawing from research by Dr. Nicholas A. Christakis and Dr. James H. Fowler, to illuminate the profound impact of social connections and the importance of surrounding yourself with positive people.[287] [288]

[286] Ruby, M. B., et al., "Vegetarianism. A Blossoming Field of Study," *Appetite*, 2013.

Social Contagion

Groundbreaking studies by Dr. Christakis and Dr. Fowler have explored the phenomenon of social contagion, revealing how behaviors and attitudes spread within social networks. Their research underscores the influential nature of social connections on individual well-being. [289] [290]

Positive emotions, attitudes, and behaviors exhibit contagious dynamics within social circles. Individuals tend to mirror and adopt the emotional states and behaviors of those around them. This phenomenon extends to happiness, optimism, and other positive attributes, emphasizing the potent impact of positive social environments on individual mindset and overall well-being.

The Neurobiology of Social Connection

Neurobiological investigations into social connections highlight the complex interplay between the brain and social interactions. The release of neurotransmitters, such as oxytocin and dopamine, is influenced by positive social experiences, contributing to feelings of connection and well-being. [291]

Studies have demonstrated that individuals with strong social support networks tend to experience lower levels of stress and exhibit better mental health outcomes. The neurobiological responses to positive social interactions contribute to a cascade of physiological benefits, underscoring the profound influence of social connections on overall health.

As you explore the importance of surrounding yourself with positive people further, you will find that the scientific evidence accentuates the role of social environments as powerful determinants of individual well-being.

---

[287] Christakis, N. A., & Fowler, J. H., "The Spread of Obesity in a Large Social Network Over 32 Years," *New England Journal of Medicine,* 2007.
[288] Christakis, N. A., & Fowler, J. H., "The Collective Dynamics of Smoking in a Large Social Network," *New England Journal of Medicine,* 2008.
[289] Christakis, N. A., & Fowler, J. H., "The Spread of Obesity in a Large Social Network Over 32 Years," ibid.
[290] Christakis, N. A., & Fowler, J. H., "The Collective Dynamics of Smoking in a Large Social Network," ibid.
[291] Insel, T. R., & Young, L. J., "The Neurobiology of Attachment," *Nature Reviews Neuroscience,* 2001.

Basically, choosing positive social connections aligns with a broader strategy you can follow for cultivating a positive mindset and fostering longevity.

CHAPTER 11: PURPOSE, MEANING, AND FULFILLMENT

INTRODUCTION

When it comes to extending longevity, the role of purpose and fulfillment emerges as a transformative force that extends beyond mere existence. This chapter explores

the profound connection between one's sense of purpose, the meaning you derive from life, and the pursuit of activities that bring fulfillment, exploring the scientific underpinnings and the impact on overall well-being and longevity.

The quest for longevity intertwines with the pursuit of purpose, a concept deeply embedded in psychological research. Dr. Viktor Frankl's seminal work on logotherapy emphasizes the significance of finding meaning in life as a driving force for human fulfillment and resilience.[292] This section navigates the pathways to discovering one's sense of purpose, drawing insights from contemporary psychologists and their research on the detailed interaction between purpose and well-being.[293]

Scientific studies, including those by Dr. Mihaly Csikszentmihalyi, reveal the transformative power of engaging in activities that foster a state of flow—immersive experiences that bring deep satisfaction and fulfillment.[294] This section explores the science behind fulfilling activities and their implications for mental and emotional well-being.

Understanding the profound connection between longevity and life's meaning involves delving into philosophical and psychological perspectives. Research by Dr. Carol Ryff and Dr. Corey L. M. Keyes sheds light on the

---

[292] Frankl, V. E., "Man's Search for Meaning," Beacon Press, 1959.

[293] Steger, M. F., et al. "The Meaning in Life Questionnaire: Assessing the Presence of and Search for Meaning in Life," *Journal of Counseling Psychology*, 2006.

[294] Csikszentmihalyi, M., "Flow: The Psychology of Optimal Experience," Harper & Row, 1990.

concept of eudaimonic well-being, emphasizing the importance of living a life rich in purpose, self-realization, and personal growth.[295] This section unveils the significance of deriving meaning from life for sustained well-being.

Scientific literature, including the works of Dr. Patricia Boyle and Dr. Nicholas T. Bott, offers insights into the relationship between a strong sense of purpose and increased longevity.[296] This final section explores the empirical evidence supporting the notion that a life imbued with purpose not only enhances the quality of existence but also contributes to a longer and healthier lifespan.

As you start your exploration of this chapter, prepare to navigate the realms of psychological, philosophical, and scientific dimensions to unravel the profound impact of purpose, meaning, and fulfillment on human longevity.

PARTICIPATING IN FULFILLING ACTIVITIES

The cultivation of a purposeful and fulfilling life extends beyond theoretical concepts to the tangible realm of daily activities and engagements. Scientific inquiry into the relationship between engaging activities and well-being reinforces the idea that the pursuit of purpose often manifests through active participation in meaningful endeavors.

Psychological theories, such as Self-Determination Theory (SDT) by Deci and Ryan, emphasize the importance of autonomy, competence, and relatedness in fostering a sense of fulfillment. Engaging in activities that align with personal values and passions promotes intrinsic motivation, contributing to a deeper sense of purpose.[297]

Research in positive psychology further substantiates the link between engaging activities and well-being. Studies exploring the concept of "positive affective events" highlight that individuals experience heightened

---

[295] Ryff, C. D., & Keyes, C. L. M. "The Structure of Psychological Well-Being Revisited," *Journal of Personality and Social Psychology*, 1995.

[296] Boyle, P. A., et al. "Effect of a Purpose in Life on Risk of Incident Alzheimer Disease and Mild Cognitive Impairment in Community-Dwelling Older Persons," *Archives of General Psychiatry*, 2009.

[297] Deci, E. L., & Ryan, R. M. "Intrinsic Motivation and Self-Determination in Human Behavior," Plenum Press, 1985.

well-being when participating in activities that bring joy, satisfaction, and a sense of accomplishment.[298]

Moreover, the notion of "flow," introduced by Csikszentmihalyi, underscores the idea that immersive and challenging activities can lead to a state of optimal experience. When individuals lose themselves in activities that align with their skills and interests, a profound sense of fulfillment emerges.[299]

Practical examples abound, ranging from pursuing hobbies, volunteering, to actively participating in one's community. The significance lies not only in the nature of the activities but in the alignment of these activities with one's values and sense of purpose.

Engaging in fulfilling activities is a pivotal component of the path toward a purposeful life. The pursuit of activities that align with personal values and passions not only contributes to immediate satisfaction but also plays a profound role in shaping an individual's overall sense of purpose and well-being.

The Nature of Fulfilling Activities

Fulfilling activities are those that resonate with an individual's intrinsic values and interests. The concept draws from the self-determination theory of Deci and Ryan which posits that activities aligned with one's internal motivations foster a sense of autonomy, competence, and relatedness.[300] This alignment is the key to experiencing deep and lasting fulfillment.

The spectrum of fulfilling activities is broad and varies from person to person. For some, it might involve creative pursuits such as art, music, or writing. For others, it could be contributing to community initiatives, engaging in meaningful work, or nurturing personal relationships. The

---

[298] Lyubomirsky, S., & Layous, K. "How Do Simple Positive Activities Increase Well-Being?," *Current Directions in Psychological Science*, 2013.

[299] Csikszentmihalyi, M., "Flow: The Psychology of Optimal Experience," Harper & Row, 1990.

[300] Deci, E. L., & Ryan, R. M., "Intrinsic Motivation and Self-Determination in Human Behavior," Springer, 1985.

[301] Csikszentmihalyi, M., "Flow: The Psychology of Optimal Experience," Harper & Row, 1990.

common thread is the alignment of these activities with an individual's values, providing a sense of purposeful engagement.

Psychological Benefits of Engagement

The psychological benefits of participating in fulfilling activities are multifaceted. Research, such as that conducted by Csikszentmihalyi on the concept of "flow," suggests that engaging in activities that challenge and stretch one's skills can lead to a state of optimal experience.[301]

This state, known as flow, is characterized by deep concentration, a sense of timelessness, and immense satisfaction. Moreover, the pursuit of fulfilling activities has been associated with increased positive affect and a reduced risk of mental health issues.

Regular engagement in activities that bring joy and satisfaction contributes to a positive emotional state, fostering resilience in the face of life's challenges.

Enhancing Well-Being through Meaningful Pursuits

Participating in fulfilling activities contributes to an individual's overall well-being. The pursuit of activities that hold personal significance adds a layer of meaning to daily life, creating an interconnected variety of experiences that contribute to an overall sense of fulfillment.

The significance of these activities extends beyond immediate gratification. Long-term engagement in pursuits aligned with one's values and passions has been linked to positive health outcomes, including lower levels of stress and a decreased risk of burnout.

The positive impact on mental and emotional well-being further underscores the importance of weaving these activities into the fabric of daily life.

Overall, the pursuit of a purposeful and fulfilling life involves a proactive engagement in activities that resonate with personal values, provide a sense of competence, and foster positive emotions. This exploration is a dynamic process, evolving as individuals grow, learn, and adapt to the changing patterns of their lives.

As you navigate the vast sea of opportunities available to you in life, the realization of your purpose in being here often unfolds through the active participation in endeavors that bring intrinsic joy and contribute to your overall well-being.

DISCOVERING YOUR SENSE OF PURPOSE

Understanding the connection between longevity and purpose necessitates an exploration into the realms of psychology, philosophy, and scientific inquiry. The pursuit of a meaningful life, as advocated by existential psychologist Dr. Viktor Frankl, serves as a cornerstone in understanding how a defined sense of purpose can significantly impact one's well-being and, ultimately, their lifespan.[302]

Recent research in positive psychology has underscored the importance of purpose as a fundamental element of psychological well-being. Studies, such as those by Steger and colleagues, have contributed to the development of tools like the Meaning in Life Questionnaire, aiding in the assessment of the presence and search for meaning in individuals' lives.[303]

The profound interplay between purpose and well-being is not merely theoretical; it finds empirical support in the field of positive psychology. The works of psychologists like Carol Ryff and Corey L. M. Keyes have researched the eudaimonic concept of well-being, emphasizing that a life rich in purpose, self-realization, and personal growth is essential for the overall flourishing of a human being.[304]

As individuals start the process of discovering their sense of purpose, engagement in activities that align with personal values and aspirations becomes paramount. Drawing insights from Csikszentmihalyi's concept of "flow" where individuals experience deep satisfaction and immersion in their pursuits reinforces the idea that purposeful activities contribute to a sense of fulfillment.[305]

---

[302] Frankl, V. E., "Man's Search for Meaning," Beacon Press, 1959.

[303] Steger, M. F., et al. "The Meaning in Life Questionnaire: Assessing the Presence of and Search for Meaning in Life," *Journal of Counseling Psychology*, 2006.

[304] Ryff, C. D., & Keyes, C. L. M. "The Structure of Psychological Well-Being Revisited," *Journal of Personality and Social Psychology*, 1995.

[305] Csikszentmihalyi, M., "Flow: The Psychology of Optimal Experience," Harper & Row, 1990.

In essence, the exploration of discovering one's sense of purpose delves into the rich variety of psychological theories, empirical research, and practical strategies. The path that leads towards longevity intertwines with the quest for a purposeful existence, making this exploration a pivotal step in understanding the dynamics of living a fulfilling life.

This study is not only a profound philosophical endeavor but also a critical aspect of health and longevity. Understanding how the discovery of purpose influences various dimensions of well-being sheds light on its significance.

A Sense of Purpose Enhances Psychological Well-Being

Discovering a sense of purpose is intrinsically tied to psychological well-being. Research, such as the work by Ryff and Singer, emphasizes the positive impact of purpose on mental health and life satisfaction.[306] Individuals who articulate a clear sense of purpose often experience lower levels of psychological distress and higher overall life satisfaction.

The process of discovering one's purpose involves introspection, self-reflection, and a deep exploration of personal values and passions. Psychological theories, including self-determination theory (Deci & Ryan, 1985), suggest that aligning one's goals and activities with intrinsic values fosters a sense of autonomy and fulfillment.[307] This alignment is a fundamental component of the path toward discovering purpose in life.

Physiological Benefits of Living a Purposeful Life

The connection between purpose and physiological health has become a subject of increasing interest in scientific inquiry. Studies, such as those conducted by Boyle et al., have identified associations between a sense of purpose and markers of physical health, including cardiovascular health.[308] Individuals with a strong sense of purpose may experience lower blood pressure, reduced inflammation, and even a lower risk of cardiovascular events.

---

[306] Ryff, C. D., & Singer, B., "The Contours of Positive Human Health," *Psychological Inquiry*, 1998.

[307] Deci, E. L., & Ryan, R. M., "Intrinsic Motivation and Self-Determination in Human Behavior," Springer, 1985.

[308] Boyle, P. A., et al., "Purpose in Life Is Associated With Mortality Among Community-Dwelling Older Persons," *Psychosomatic Medicine*, 2009.

The physiological benefits of purpose may be linked to stress reduction. Purposeful individuals often exhibit lower cortisol levels, indicating a more balanced stress response. Additionally, purposeful living has been correlated with improved sleep patterns, further contributing to overall health.

Longevity and Purpose

The impact of purpose on longevity is a subject that has garnered attention in the field of positive psychology. Research, such as the longitudinal study by Hill and Turiano, has shown that individuals with a sense of purpose tend to live longer lives.[309]

This association may be attributed to the various positive health outcomes linked to purpose, from healthier lifestyle choices to enhanced resilience in the face of life's challenges.

The path to discovering one's sense of purpose is an ongoing process that involves self-discovery, growth, and adaptation. It is a dynamic aspect of the human experience that unfolds across the lifespan, influencing both immediate well-being and the trajectory of one's overall health.

DERIVING MEANING FROM LIFE

The quest for a purposeful existence often intersects with the profound pursuit of meaning in life. Scholars and researchers from various disciplines have studied the multifaceted nature of meaning, offering insights into how individuals derive profound significance from their experiences and contributions.

Victor Frankl, a psychiatrist and Holocaust survivor, explored the essence of finding meaning even in the darkest moments in his seminal work from 1959 entitled "Man's Search for Meaning". His existential analysis emphasizes the human capacity to derive meaning through enduring suffering and choosing one's response to life's challenges.

Existential psychologists, such as Yalom and Batthyany, have extended Frankl's work by highlighting the importance of personal responsibility and the search for meaning as fundamental aspects of human existence.[310] Their

---

[309] Hill, P. L., & Turiano, N. A., "Purpose in Life as a Predictor of Mortality Across Adulthood," *Psychological Science*, 2014.

contributions underscore the idea that meaning is not merely discovered but actively constructed through a purposeful engagement with life.

Positive psychology research, spearheaded by scholars like Seligman and Steger, has furthered the exploration of meaning and its association with well-being. Steger's Meaning in Life Questionnaire (MLQ) has become a widely used instrument for assessing the various dimensions of meaning, emphasizing the significance of purpose and coherence in one's life.[311] [312]

In practical terms, individuals often derive meaning from various sources, including relationships, work, creativity, and contribution to society. Volunteering, pursuing passions, and engaging in activities aligned with personal values emerge as pathways to a more meaningful life.[313]

In conclusion, the shift towards finding purpose and fulfillment in life intertwines with the profound search for meaning. From existential reflections to contemporary positive psychology, a rich variety of insights provides guidance on how you can actively construct and derive profound significance from your existence that will in turn likely extend your life.

A Profound Impact on Well-Being

The pursuit of meaning in life is a fundamental aspect of the human experience, and its implications for overall well-being and longevity are profound.

Understanding how deriving meaning from life contributes to these outcomes involves exploring psychological, physiological, and behavioral dimensions.

Psychological Resilience

One of the key psychological benefits associated with deriving meaning from life is increased resilience in the face of adversity. Research, such as

---

[310] Yalom, I. D., "Existential Psychotherapy," Basic Books, 1980.

[311] Seligman, M. E., "Authentic Happiness," Free Press, 2002.

[312] Steger, M. F., "Meaning in Life: A Brief Introduction," Wiley, 2020.

[313] Ryff, C. D., & Singer, B. H., "Know Thyself and Become What You Are: A Eudaimonic Approach to Psychological Well-Being," *Journal of Happiness Studies*, 2008.

that conducted by Park and Folkman, highlights the role of meaning-making in coping with life stressors.[314]

Individuals who find meaning in challenging circumstances tend to exhibit greater psychological resilience, navigating difficulties with a sense of purpose and coherence.

Meaning-making can involve the reinterpretation of experiences, finding purpose in adversity, and deriving a sense of personal growth from challenges.

This psychological resilience, in turn, contributes to lower levels of stress and improved mental health, factors that have been linked to enhanced longevity.

Neurobiological Correlates

The exploration of meaning and its neural correlates has garnered attention in neuroscientific research. Neurobiological studies, including those by Kringelbach and Berridge, suggest that experiences related to meaning and purpose may activate reward circuits in the brain.[315] This activation can lead to the release of neurochemicals associated with pleasure and well-being, contributing to an overall positive mood.

Moreover, the neurobiological impact of meaning extends beyond immediate emotional states. Long-term engagement with meaningful activities may influence brain plasticity and neurogenesis, potentially promoting cognitive health and resilience to age-related cognitive decline.

Behavioral Health Choices

Deriving meaning from life often shapes individuals' behavioral choices, particularly in areas related to health and self-care. Meaningful pursuits are frequently associated with a sense of responsibility towards one's well-being and the well-being of others.

---

[314] Park, C. L., & Folkman, S., "Meaning in the Context of Stress and Coping," *Review of General Psychology*, 1997.
[315] Kringelbach, M. L., & Berridge, K. C., "Towards a Functional Neuroanatomy of Pleasure and Happiness," *Trends in Cognitive Sciences*, 2009.

This sense of responsibility can manifest in healthier lifestyle choices, including regular exercise, balanced nutrition, and avoidance of harmful habits.

Studies, such as those by Steptoe and Fancourt, highlight the positive impact of engaging in cultural and artistic activities, which often contribute to a sense of meaning, on overall well-being and longevity. [316] These activities not only provide enjoyment but also serve as outlets for creative expression and a source of purpose.

In essence, deriving meaning from life is a multifaceted phenomenon with implications for mental, neurological, and behavioral dimensions. It fosters psychological resilience, activates rewarding neural pathways, and guides individuals towards choices that support both their immediate well-being and long-term health.

CONNECTING PURPOSE TO LONGEVITY

The exploration of purpose and its potential impact on longevity has garnered attention from researchers investigating the detailed links between mental well-being and physical health. Numerous studies underscore the potential health benefits associated with a sense of purpose, suggesting that individuals with a clear purpose may experience enhanced overall well-being.

In a longitudinal study conducted by Boyle et al., it was found that a higher sense of purpose in life was associated with a reduced risk of mortality among older adults.[317] The research indicated that individuals with a stronger sense of purpose exhibited a survival advantage over those with a weaker sense of purpose, emphasizing the potential role of purpose in promoting longevity.

---

[316] Steptoe, A., & Fancourt, D., "Cultural Engagement and Mental Health: Does Enjoying Cultural Activities Predict Better Mental Health in Older Age?" *The British Journal of Psychiatry*, 2019.
[317] Boyle, P. A., Barnes, L. L., Buchman, A. S., & Bennett, D. A., "Purpose in Life Is Associated With Mortality Among Community-Dwelling Older Persons," *Psychosomatic Medicine*, 2010.

Furthermore, research in the field of psychoneuroimmunology has explored how psychological factors, including a sense of purpose, may influence the immune system.

Studies, such as those by Segerstrom and Miller, suggest that positive psychological states, which can be fostered by a sense of purpose, may contribute to improved immune functioning.[318]

The mechanisms underlying the connection between purpose and longevity are complex and multifaceted. One plausible explanation involves the stress-buffering effects of purpose, as individuals with a strong sense of purpose may be more resilient in the face of life's challenges, potentially mitigating the physiological impact of stress.

In summary, the intersection of purpose and longevity unveils a fascinating interplay between psychological well-being and physical health. While more research is needed to fully elucidate the mechanisms involved, the existing evidence suggests that cultivating a sense of purpose may contribute to a longer and healthier life.

Unveiling the Mechanisms

The intriguing link between a sense of purpose and longevity highlights the complex mechanisms that underscore the relationship between mental outlook and physical health.

While research has established a correlation, understanding how purpose exerts its influence on longevity requires a closer examination of the underlying processes.

Stress-Buffering Effects

One of the primary mechanisms through which a sense of purpose may contribute to longevity is by acting as a buffer against stress. Stress, a pervasive aspect of modern life, is known to have detrimental effects on both mental and physical health.

---

[318] Segerstrom, S. C., & Miller, G. E., "Psychological Stress and the Human Immune System: A Meta-Analytic Study of 30 Years of Inquiry," *Psychological Bulletin*, 2004.

Individuals with a strong sense of purpose may exhibit greater resilience in the face of stressors, thereby minimizing the physiological toll that chronic stress can take on the body.

Studies, such as those by Ryff and Singer, have explored how purpose in life can moderate the impact of stress on health outcomes.[319] The stress-buffering effects of purpose may involve psychological processes that help individuals reframe challenges, maintain a positive outlook, and cope more effectively with adversity.

Psychoneuroimmunology Insights

The burgeoning field of psychoneuroimmunology has provided additional insights into the ways in which psychological states, including a sense of purpose, can influence the immune system.

The immune system plays a key role in defending the body against pathogens and maintaining overall health. Positive psychological factors, such as purpose, may contribute to enhanced immune functioning, potentially reducing the risk of illness and promoting longevity.

Studies, including those by Cohen et al., have explored how positive psychological states can influence immune responses.[320] While the exact mechanisms are still being elucidated, it is hypothesized that the psychosocial resources associated with a sense of purpose may contribute to a more robust and responsive immune system.

Healthier Lifestyles

Another facet of the connection between purpose and longevity may involve the adoption of healthier lifestyles and lifestyle factors like favoring a plant-based diet.

Individuals with a clear sense of purpose often report a higher level of motivation and engagement in activities that contribute to their well-being. This can include maintaining a balanced plant-based diet, engaging in regular physical activity, and avoiding harmful behaviors.

---

[319] Ryff, C. D., & Singer, B., "The Contours of Positive Human Health," Psychological Inquiry, 1998.
[320] Cohen, S., Alper, C. M., Doyle, W. J., Adler, N., Treanor, J. J., & Turner, R. B., "Objective and Subjective Socioeconomic Status and Susceptibility to the Common Cold," *Health Psychology*, 2008.

Research by Kim et al. suggests that purpose in life is associated with a reduced risk of developing chronic diseases, potentially due to the adoption of healthier lifestyles.[321] The motivation derived from a sense of purpose may empower individuals to make choices that support their long-term health, indirectly influencing their lifespan.

In essence, the interplay between purpose and longevity is a dynamic and evolving field of study. While stress buffering, psychoneuroimmunology, and healthier lifestyles offer insights into the potential mechanisms, ongoing research is essential to unravel the full complexity of this intriguing connection.

---

[321] Kim, E. S., Sun, J. K., Park, N., & Peterson, C., "Purpose in Life and Reduced Risk of Myocardial Infarction Among Older U.S. Adults With Coronary Heart Disease: A Two-Year Follow-Up," *Journal of Behavioral Medicine*, 2013.

CONCLUSION

CONCLUSION

In the culminating chapter of this comprehensive guide to longevity and well-being, you will now come to the end of our journey together, synthesizing the secrets that will unveil the pathway to a long and healthy life as you put them into practice.

Grounded in scientific principles and evidence, the two key sections of this concluding chapter will serve as a compass for integrating the knowledge gleaned throughout this book into actionable steps for a robust and resilient future.

This concluding chapter aims to help you amalgamate the various insights garnered from this book that were based on extensive research, authoritative studies, and the collective wisdom of experts in the fields of nutrition, exercise, stress management, substance use habits, sleep quality, social connections, mental well-being, and purposeful living.

Drawing from the wealth of scientific literature on the subject of health and longevity presented earlier in this book, this concluding chapter aims to distill and summarize the key principles, secrets and factors that contribute to a enjoying prolonged and thriving life.

THE SECRETS TO A LONG AND HEALTHY LIFE

In this book's science-based exploration of longevity, you have seen how to start leading a robust and enduring life, drawing from a wealth of scientific evidence, authoritative studies, and expert insights.

As you start to synthesize and apply in your daily life the secrets to a long and healthy existence that you have learned in the previous chapters of this book, it should become increasingly evident that a multifaceted approach, encompassing various aspects of lifestyle and health, will contribute best to your overall well-being.

This section contains a brief summary of the key teachings of each chapter of this book to aid your synthesis of this information so you can better integrate it into your life going forward.

Follow a Nutrient-Rich Diet

As laid out in detail in the first chapter of this book, the best and most natural nutrition suitable for your great ape physiology forms the cornerstone of optimal health.

Research by Drs. Ornish, Lindeberg, Esselstyn, and Campbell underscores the pivotal role of a raw and nutrient-rich plant-based diet in preventing chronic diseases and ensuring optimal vitality well into your golden years. [322]

Balance Your Plate Properly

When embracing a plant-centric dietary approach, how you balance your plate matters. Focusing mainly on raw fruits and greens, along with lesser amounts of vegetables, whole grains, legumes, nuts, and seeds, has been associated with improved blood glucose concentrations, body weight, lipid profiles, and blood pressure.[323]

To enjoy those health benefits, this chapter promoted a dietary ratio of 50% fruit, 40% greens, and 10% other foods. This proportion is based on the scientific concept of physiological diet derived from observing the foods that similar great ape populations living wild naturally select.

These dietary percentages emerge as a compelling guide to optimal health and align with scientific evidence suggesting that such a diet can have a very positive impact on cardiovascular health, weight management, vitality, immune function, sugar metabolism, and overall longevity. [324]

---

[322] Ornish, D., Lindeberg, S., Esselstyn, C., & Campbell, T., "Nutritional and Lifestyle Guidelines for the Prevention of Cardiovascular Disease." *The American Journal of Cardiology*, 82(2), 138-143, 2009.

[323] Harvard T.H. Chan School of Public Health. (2012). "The Nutrition Source." Retrieved from https://www.hsph.harvard.edu/nutritionsource/

[324] Fuhrman, J., (2011) "The End of Diabetes" and (2021) "Eat for Life", HarperOne.

[325] National Institute on Aging. (2017). "Aging Hearts and Arteries: A Scientific Quest." Retrieved from https://www.nia.nih.gov/

Make Exercise Your Lifelong Companion

Having explained the importance of getting regular exercise in Chapter 3, you should now see that the marriage of cardiovascular and strength training can play a pivotal role in moving your body towards a healthier and longer life.

Scientific studies emphasize the positive impact of regular physical activity on various facets of health, from cardiovascular function to cognitive well-being. [325]

Furthermore, finding happiness in getting exercise will serve you well in life, since you will enjoy engaging in the exact process that makes and keeps you healthier.

Enjoy Quality Sleep

In Chapter 4, you learned about the secrets of unlocking a restful night, and how important maintaining healthy sleep habits is to your overall health and longevity.

From the regulation of metabolic functions to the enhancement of cognitive abilities, quality sleep emerges as a cornerstone of longevity.

Use Stress Management Techniques

From reading Chapter 5, you have gained an understanding of the impact of stress on your health. Practicing mindfulness and meditation, and developing resilience collectively form a robust toolkit for navigating life's challenges.

Scientifically validated strategies presented earlier in this book can help mitigate the detrimental effects of chronic stress, contributing to your overall well-being.

Form Social Connections

In Chapter 6, the importance of social connection factor to longevity was explored in detail. This study demonstrated the profound impact that interpersonal relationships can have on your overall well-being.

Delving into the science-backed reasons for building strong relationships shows how positive social interactions can influence your mental health for the better. In doing so, you learned how finding support and joy in social connections generally plays a pivotal role in fostering psychological resilience and enhancing the overall quality of life.

Learning from authoritative studies on the topic, you gained valuable insights into the detailed dynamics that make social bonds integral to the pursuit of longevity.

Break Harmful Habits

Chapter 7 offered a comprehensive guide to liberating yourself from detrimental lifestyle choices that will very likely shorten your lifespan.

If you drink alcohol, start this process by directly addressing the harms of alcohol intake, including the adverse health effects and societal consequences of excessive alcohol consumption. If you smoke tobacco or use harmful drugs, it also makes sense to resolve to commence the challenging process of quitting smoking and such drug use to enjoy better health results over time.

Finally, overcoming physiological addictions offers considerable longevity benefits. Following evidence-based methods and strategies to end drug addictions can empower you in your pursuit of a thriving and substance-free life.

Get Regular Checkups

Chapter 8 placed a strong emphasis on proactive health management. This process of taking charge of your own well-being strengthens as you grasp the significance of monitoring your health, deriving benefits that include the early detection and prevention of troublesome diseases that are expensive to treat and may cost you your life and/or its quality.

Looking at maintaining your health through a collaborative lens, you were encouraged to engage with healthcare professionals actively to create a symbiotic relationship aimed at optimizing your well-being.

Grounded in scientific principles, this chapter served as a practical guide to navigating the healthcare landscape. It also underscored the importance of undertaking regular check-ups on your path toward a healthier and longer life.

With that noted, some studies do caution against the excessive use of radiation-based early detection screening techniques, such as x-rays and mammograms, due to the potential cancer risks.

Pursue Lifelong Learning

In Chapter 9, the practice of continuously engaging in the learning process over your lifetime was shown to offer considerable longevity benefits that stand as a testament to the great value of intellectual stimulation.

By stimulating the mind in ways that tend to prolong longevity, the role of continuous learning and growth in promoting cognitive health becomes increasingly clear. As you explore the symbiotic link between intellectual stimulation and overall well-being further going forward, it makes good sense to integrate stimulating and strategic intellectual activities into your daily life.

With a focus on the transformative potential of engaging in a lifelong learning mindset, you now have a roadmap for enhancing your mental acuity in order to live a more fulfilling and enduring life with a sharper and clearer mind.

Cultivate a Positive Mindset

Chapter 10 immersed you in the transformative power of positivity. From understanding the intrinsic influence of positivity to delving into the value of affirmations and prayer, you were offered evidence-based insights into the value of fostering optimism and gratitude.

You also explored the mind-body connection and its notable impact on health, which unveiled the profound impact of maintaining a positive mindset on your overall well-being.

By emphasizing the importance of surrounding oneself with positive influences, this chapter stands as as a guide for those seeking to harness the inherent connection between a favorable mental outlook and longevity.

Finding Purpose, Meaning and Fulfillment

The penultimate chapter of this book focused on finding purpose, meaning, and fulfillment in life. The discussion regarding performing this profound task explored the key elements that give life meaning.

By discovering your own unique sense of purpose and meaning in life, you can start to experience the transformative potential of participating in fulfilling activities that align with your purpose.

Engaging in this introspective process can in turn highlight the deep connection between deriving meaning from life and how that contributes to your overall well-being. Consider exploring the importance to your longevity of first connecting to your life's purpose and then furthering it as you live.

Putting these ideas into practice can help you attain a higher and more holistic point of view regarding your life. Having a sense of purpose in life can truly serve as a guiding force toward a more fulfilling and enduring existence.

FINAL THOUGHTS

The key insights and techniques in this book are grounded in rigorous scientific inquiry. Taken seriously and implemented as part of a general longevity program, they offer a comprehensive guide to the interconnected secrets of living a prolonged and healthy life.

As you move forward, keep in mind that a lifelong process is best seen from a holistic lens since it encompasses various aspects of physical, mental, and emotional well-being. This book has aimed to guide you through these key components in a manner grounded in science, emphasizing the essential significance of good nutrition while also addressing other key lifestyle factors that contribute to long term well-being.

Building upon the synthesized insights from this book, you are now encouraged to translate the knowledge you have gained into tangible steps you can take if you are seeking a proactive approach to securing a healthier and more vibrant future.

By keeping your focus on pragmatic strategies grounded in scientific understanding, you can henceforth implement the actionable measures propounded in this book in your daily life. Embarking on this process will empower you to take charge of your well-being so that you can walk a healthier path and enjoy a longer life.

As this exploration into the science-backed principles of a flourishing life concludes, the synthesis of knowledge and actionable steps in this book are intended to serve as a beacon. May it guide you towards a brighter future characterized by vitality, resilience, and enduring well-being.

Furthermore, by transitioning from absorbing the lessons of this book to actively engaging in the practical application of the key secrets it contains, may you feel increasingly empowered to embark on a path of personal transformation towards better health and enhanced longevity.

148

APPENDICES

APPENDIX A: FURTHER READING

The high quality resources listed below provide in-depth insights and complement the information presented in this book, offering a broader understanding of the multifaceted aspects of achieving a long and healthy life.

1. **Nutrition and Longevity:**
   - *Eat to Live* by Joel Fuhrman, M.D.
   - *The End of Diabetes* by Joel Fuhrman, M.D.
   - *How Not to Die* by Michael Greger, M.D.
   - *How to Survive a Pandemic* by Michael Greger, M.D.
2. **Physical Fitness and Longevity:**
   - *The China Study* by T. Colin Campbell, Ph.D., and Thomas M. Campbell II, M.D.
   - *Spark: The Revolutionary New Science of Exercise and the Brain* by John J. Ratey, M.D.
3. **Quality Sleep and Longevity:**
   - *Why We Sleep: Unlocking the Power of Sleep and Dreams* by Matthew Walker, Ph.D.
4. **Stress Management:**
   - *The Relaxation Response* by Herbert Benson, M.D.
   - *Full Catastrophe Living* by Jon Kabat-Zinn, Ph.D.
5. **Social Connections and Well-Being:**
   - *The Loneliness Cure* by Kory Floyd, Ph.D.
   - *Connected: The Surprising Power of Our Social Networks and How They Shape Our Lives* by Nicholas A. Christakis, M.D., Ph.D., and James H. Fowler, Ph.D.
6. **Substance Use and Addiction:**
   - *The Biology of Desire: Why Addiction Is Not a Disease* by Marc Lewis, Ph.D.
7. **Health Check-ups and Preventive Medicine:**
   - *The Patient Will See You Now: The Future of Medicine is in Your Hands* by Eric Topol, M.D.
8. **Lifelong Learning and Cognitive Health:**

- *The Brain That Changes Itself* by Norman Doidge, M.D.
- *Make It Stick: The Science of Successful Learning* by Peter C. Brown, Henry L. Roediger III, and Mark A. McDaniel.

9. **Positive Mindset and Well-Being:**
- *Learned Optimism: How to Change Your Mind and Your Life* by Martin E.P. Seligman, Ph.D.
- *The How of Happiness: A New Approach to Getting the Life You Want* by Sonja Lyubomirsky, Ph.D.

10. **Purpose and Fulfillment:**
- *Man's Search for Meaning* by Viktor E. Frankl, M.D., Ph.D.
- *Drive: The Surprising Truth About What Motivates Us* by Daniel H. Pink.

11. **Comprehensive Health and Longevity:**
- *The Blue Zones: Lessons for Living Longer from the People Who've Lived the Longest* by Dan Buettner.

12. **Official Reports and Guidelines:**
- World Health Organization (WHO) Reports on Healthy Living and Longevity.
- Centers for Disease Control and Prevention (CDC) Guidelines on Preventive Health Measures.

APPENDIX B: A WEEK OF SAMPLE MEAL PLANS

The following seven sample meal plans are designed to cover a full week time frame and provide a balanced, raw, plant-based diet aiming for around 2,000 calories per day. In general, these plans prioritize a distribution of 50% fruit, 40% leafy greens, and 10% other plant-based foods, which corresponds to the dietary ratios most suitable for the human physiology.

The sample meal plans listed below provide a glimpse into a raw, plant-based diet focused on achieving a balance of essential nutrients and promoting overall health, vitality and youthfulness. To personalize these plans, you can adjust portion sizes based on your individual caloric needs and weight management goals, and the dishes based on your personal food preferences.

Day 1:
1. **Breakfast:**
   - *Smoothie Bowl:* Blend berries, banana, and spinach. Top with chia seeds and sliced kiwi.
2. **Lunch:**
   - *Large Salad:* Mix kale, arugula, tomatoes, cucumber, and avocado. Dress with lemon-tahini dressing.
3. **Snack:**
   - *Fresh Fruit Platter:* Assorted seasonal fruits (e.g., pears, pineapple, berries, and mango).
4. **Dinner:**
   - *Zucchini Noodles with Pesto:* Spiralize zucchini and toss with a raw basil and walnut basil pesto.

Day 2:
1. **Breakfast:**
   - *Green Smoothie:* Blend spinach, kale, apple, and pear with a splash of coconut water.
2. **Lunch:**

- *Nori Rolls:* Fill raw nori sheets with julienned vegetables, avocado, and sprouts. Serve with almond dipping sauce.

3. **Snack:**
    - *Mixed Berries and Almonds:* Handful of berries with a side of raw almonds.

4. **Dinner:**
    - *Rainbow Salad:* Combine shredded beets, carrots, and cabbage. Add mixed greens and top with a citrus vinaigrette.

Day 3:

1. **Breakfast:**
    - *Fruit Salad:* Mix melon, grapes, and citrus fruits. Sprinkle with chopped mint.

2. **Lunch:**
    - *Collard Wraps:* Fill collard green leaves with hummus, shredded carrots, cucumber, and avocado.

3. **Snack:**
    - *Mango Slices with Chili Powder:* Fresh mango slices sprinkled with a pinch of chili powder.

4. **Dinner:**
    - *Portobello Mushroom Steaks:* Marinate portobello mushrooms and serve with a side of spiralized raw zucchini.

Day 4:

1. **Breakfast:**
    - *Acai Bowl:* Blend acai berries with banana and top with raw granola, coconut flakes, and sliced strawberries.

2. **Lunch:**
    - *Cucumber Noodles with Avocado Sauce:* Spiralize a cucumber and toss with a creamy avocado and lime dressing.

3. **Snack:**
    - *Orange Slices and Walnuts:* Fresh orange slices paired with raw walnuts.

4. **Dinner:**
    - *Tomato Basil Zoodles:* Spiralized zucchini noodles with cherry tomatoes, basil, and pine nut pesto.

Day 5:

1. **Breakfast:**
    - *Pineapple-Mint Smoothie:* Blend pineapple, mint, and coconut water for a refreshing smoothie.

2. **Lunch:**
   - *Spinach and Strawberry Salad:* Combine baby spinach, sliced strawberries, and raw soaked sunflower seeds. Dress with balsamic vinaigrette.
3. **Snack:**
   - *Grape and Walnut Medley:* Red and green grapes with raw walnuts.
4. **Dinner:**
   - *Cabbage Leaf Tacos:* Fill cabbage leaves with seasoned walnut "meat" made with sundried tomatoes, topped with salsa, and guacamole.

Day 6:

1. **Breakfast:**
   - *Mango-Papaya Smoothie:* Blend mango, papaya, and a splash of coconut water.
2. **Lunch:**
   - *Rainbow Veggie Bowl:* Combine julienned bell peppers, carrots, and cherry tomatoes. Top with a zesty lemon-tahini dressing.
3. **Snack:**
   - *Kiwi and Almond Butter:* Sliced kiwi served with a side of raw almond butter.
4. **Dinner:**
   - *Raw Pad Thai:* Julienne zucchini and carrots, toss with a spicy almond butter sauce, and garnish with cilantro.

Day 7:
1. **Breakfast:**
   - *Blueberry-Chia Pudding:* Mix soaked chia seeds with coconut milk and top with fresh blueberries.
2. **Lunch:**
   - *Avocado and Tomato Salad:* Combine ripe avocado, cherry tomatoes, and arugula. Drizzle with lemon juice and cold pressed olive oil.
3. **Snack:**
   - *Banana and Walnut Bites:* Sliced bananas with a sprinkle of crushed walnuts.
4. **Dinner:**
   - *Cauliflower Rice Sushi Rolls:* Fill nori sheets with cauliflower rice, avocado, and cucumber. Serve with ginger and nama shoyu.

APPENDIX C: GLOSSARY OF RELEVANT TERMS

This glossary provides comprehensive definitions for key terms used in "The Secrets to a Long and Healthy Life" to enhance readers' understanding of the concepts presented in this book.

1. **Aerobic Exercise:** Aerobic exercise, also known as cardiovascular exercise, involves activities that increase the heart rate and improve the efficiency of the cardiovascular system. Examples include running, cycling, and swimming.
2. **Body Mass Index (BMI):** Body Mass Index is a measurement used to assess an individual's body weight in relation to their height. It is commonly employed as an indicator of whether a person has a healthy weight.
3. **Cognitive Flexibility:** Cognitive flexibility is the ability to adapt and switch between different tasks or mental processes. It plays a key role in problem-solving and navigating complex situations.
4. **Deep Breathing:** Deep breathing is a relaxation technique that involves taking slow, deliberate breaths to promote a sense of calmness and reduce stress.
5. **Essential Nutrients:** Essential nutrients are substances that the body needs to function properly but cannot produce on its own. They must be obtained through diet and include vitamins, minerals, and amino acids.
6. **Fiber:** Fiber is a type of carbohydrate found in plant-based foods. It promotes digestive health, helps control blood sugar levels, and contributes to a feeling of fullness.
7. **Holistic Health:** Holistic health considers the interconnectedness of physical, mental, and social well-being. It emphasizes addressing all aspects of an individual's health.
8. **Hypnotherapy:** Hypnotherapy is a therapeutic technique that uses hypnosis to induce a state of focused attention and heightened suggestibility. It aims to help individuals explore their thoughts, feelings, and behaviors, facilitating positive changes.
9. **Intellectual Stimulation:** Intellectual stimulation refers to activities that engage and challenge the mind, promoting cognitive

health. This can include reading, solving puzzles, and participating in activities that require continuous learning.

10. **Interval Training:** Interval training involves alternating between periods of high-intensity exercise and periods of rest or lower-intensity activity. It can enhance cardiovascular fitness and calorie burning.

11. **Joint Health:** Joint health refers to the condition of the body's joints, including the muscles, ligaments, and cartilage. Exercise and proper nutrition contribute to maintaining joint health.

12. **Lifestyle Medicine:** Lifestyle medicine focuses on addressing health issues through lifestyle interventions, including diet, exercise, stress management, and other non-pharmacological approaches.

13. **Mental Resilience:** Mental resilience involves the ability to adapt and recover from adversity, stress, or trauma, maintaining mental well-being in challenging situations.

14. **Mindfulness:** Mindfulness is a practice that involves paying attention to the present moment without judgment. It often includes techniques such as meditation and deep breathing to promote mental well-being.

15. **Neuroplasticity:** Neuroplasticity is the brain's ability to reorganize itself by forming new neural connections throughout life. It plays a role in learning, memory, and recovery from injury.

16. **Nutrient-Dense Diet:** A nutrient-dense diet focuses on foods that provide a high concentration of essential nutrients per calorie. This includes raw fruits and leafy greens, as well as vegetables, whole grains, and low-fat plant proteins.

17. **Omega-3 Fatty Acids:** Omega-3 fatty acids are essential fats that play a key role in brain function and heart health. They are commonly found in flaxseeds, hemp seeds, algal oil, and walnuts.

18. **Plant-Based Diet:** A plant-based diet emphasizes whole, plant-derived foods and limits or excludes animal products. It is associated with various health benefits, including reduced risk of chronic diseases.

19. **Quality Sleep:** Quality sleep refers to achieving restful and rejuvenating sleep, essential for physical and mental health.

20. **Raw Food Diet:** A raw food diet involves consuming only uncooked food either in its whole food form or processed directly from whole foods.

21. **Resilience:** Resilience is the ability to adapt and bounce back from challenges and adversity. It involves developing coping mechanisms and maintaining mental and emotional well-being during difficult times.

22. **Resistance Training:** Resistance training involves using external

resistance, such as weights or resistance bands, to build muscle strength and endurance.

23. **Self-Reflection:** Self-reflection is the process of examining and contemplating one's thoughts, feelings, and actions, contributing to personal growth and self-awareness.

24. **Social Connections:** Social connections refer to the relationships and interactions individuals have with others. Building strong social connections is linked to improved well-being and longevity.

25. **Strength Training:** Strength training involves exercises designed to enhance muscle strength and endurance. It includes activities such as weightlifting, resistance training, and bodyweight exercises.

26. **Stress Management:** Stress management encompasses techniques and strategies to cope with and reduce stress. This can include mindfulness, meditation, and other relaxation techniques.

27. **Substance Use Disorders:** Substance use disorders involve the harmful or hazardous use of substances, including alcohol and drugs, leading to addiction and negative health consequences.

28. **Time-Restricted Eating:** Time-restricted eating, also sometimes called intermittent fasting, is an eating pattern that involves consuming all daily calories within a specific window, often with a prolonged fasting period.

29. **UV Exposure:** UV exposure refers to exposure to ultraviolet radiation from the sun. While sunlight is a natural source of vitamin D3 for humans, excessive UV exposure can contribute to skin damage.

30. **Well-Being:** Well-being is a holistic concept that includes physical, mental, and social health. It reflects an individual's overall state of happiness and life satisfaction.

31. **Whole Foods:** Whole foods are minimally processed, unrefined, and unprocessed foods that retain their natural nutrients. Examples include fruits, leafy greens, vegetables, whole grains, and plant-derived protein sources like nuts, seeds, and legumes.

ABOUT THE AUTHOR

After obtaining her physical science degrees, Alice Dee studied nutritional healing and herbology for decades. In addition to growing a thriving food forest, she also founded a pioneering raw plant-based restaurant in Northern California. Alice is the author of numerous other books related to nutrition and plant-based diets, as well as the organizer of related online forums. Alice is available for consulting on raw, plant based diets and nutritional healing.

For more information, please visit her websites at

www.RawFromTheGarden.com

www.NutritionalHealer.com

www.PeakPerformanceDiet.com

www.TheFoodForestGuide.com

For fully raw plant-based recipes suitable for the 50-40-10 physiological diet buy Alice's restaurant-tested Raw Vegan Recipes book here:

www.RawVeganRecipesBook.com

For additional support, you can join her large and active Raw Vegan Recipes Facebook Group here:

www.facebook.com/groups/rawveganrecipes1/

www.ingramcontent.com/pod-product-compliance
Lightning Source LLC
Chambersburg PA
CBHW050727260726

48661CB00001B/98